D0094893

JEAN'S WAY

ALSO BY DEREK HUMPHRY

Because They're Black (with Gus John)
Police Power and Black People
Passports and Politics (with Michael Ward)
The Cricket Conspiracy
False Messiah: The Story of Michael X
  (with David Tindall)

JEAN'S WAY

Derek Humphry
with Ann Wickett

QUARTET BOOKS

For Roy and Sid

Copyright © 1978 by Derek Humphry and Ann Wickett

All rights reserved, including the right to reproduce this book or portions thereof in any form.

Published in the United States of America 1978 by Quartet Books Inc., a member of the Namara Group, 12 East 69 Street, New York, New York 10021.

Manufactured in the United States of America.

Library of Congress Cataloging in Publication Data

Humphry, Derek, 1930-
  Jean's way.

  1. Breast—Cancer—Biography. 2. Right to die.
3. Euthanasia. 4. Humphry, Jean. I. Wickett,
Ann, joint author. II. Title.
RC280.B8H85   362.1′9′6994490926 [B]   78-15113
ISBN 0-7043-2165-2

WIDENER UNIVERSITY
WOLFGRAM
LIBRARY
CHESTER, PA.
DISCARDED WIDENER UNIVERSITY

CONTENTS

PREFACE

The one certain thing in life is that we shall die. But how shall we cope with the process of dying? Modern science makes the end of our lives less painful physically but cannot start to deal with the emotional and spiritual problems – only the individuals concerned and their loved ones can solve these.

This account of how a couple, happily married for twenty-two years, handled their impending separation by the wife's death is, of course, highly individual. It is one way to die. The purpose of describing Jean's way is to open the debate, both within one's own mind and in the public forum, on how to die.

There is little doubt that Jean's susceptibility to the disease which killed her was hereditary. We are at a stage when cancer is slowly but surely being mastered but Jean was not one of the lucky ones. Today many cancers are entirely curable. Early detection, surgery, drugs, irradiation and immunology contain the others and offer a hopeful future.

'Cancer research has at last turned the corner and is on a winning stretch,' writes Dr Oliver Gillie, geneticist and medical correspondent of the *Sunday Times*, in his conclusion to a world survey of the battle against the disease.

Nevertheless cancer remains one of the commonest causes of death. With this cause, as with any other, let the recognition that it is inevitable be made at the right time and in an honest way so that the individual may arrange that his or her last days are spent in the happiest manner whilst the loved ones also prepare themselves for the separation and its aftermath.

Finally, I would like to add that it was entirely because Jean prepared and fortified me for her death that I never ceased believing in the power of love; thus after a year, I had met and married Ann Wickett, whose idea it was to write this book, who encouraged me during the painful moments of remembering, and assisted in the writing, editing, and typing.

Derek Humphry
London, 1977

JEAN'S WAY

1 ON HER TERMS

As I placed the breakfast tray at my wife's bedside table she looked across at me and asked, 'Is this the day?'

'Yes, my darling, it is,' I replied. I had known for some time now.

'All right,' she declared, 'I shall die at one o'clock. That's good. I'm glad it's been decided.'

I was not surprised at her statement. For two years and four months she had known she had cancer and almost a year previously we had made a pact about what to do when the end was close.

In the four hours we had left, we reviewed our twenty-two years of marriage, discussed our three children and their futures, and what would happen to me when she was dead. We reflected on the happy years of our lives together, the good decisions and the occasional bad ones.

Always of a clear mind, she reminded me that this was Easter Saturday and that Monday was a holiday as well so I would not be able to register her death until Tuesday. She gave explicit instructions about the disposal of clothing and personal effects.

We talked on until a few minutes before one o'clock when I left the room to make a hot drink. I prepared two mugs of coffee, both with milk, and into one mug I put a strong mixture of dissolved pain-killing and sleeping tablets which I knew

1

would be lethal. When I returned to her room I handed this mug to her.

'Is this it?' she asked.

She knew what it contained. We gave one another a last embrace while we said farewell. She gulped the coffee, set down the mug on the bedside table barely in time before she began to pass out, murmuring, 'Good-bye, darling.'

She fell into a deep sleep, breathing heavily. I watched over her until fifty minutes later her breathing stopped.

For several minutes I remained with her, composing my thoughts before I went to tell the children.

That Jean Humphry should die at the age of forty-two, in the bloom of life, was a great sorrow to all of us who loved her. However, having accepted that the disease was going to eventually kill her, she spent the remaining two years living such a joyful, caring, purposeful life that it mattered a good deal less that her life was shortened by twenty or thirty years. And she died on her own terms, not those of the disease which ravaged her body.

2 DISCOVERY

Just three years earlier, Jean and I had been speculating about how to spend the second half of our life together and we considered many possibilities. That August, the summer of 1972, we were able to take the first holiday since our honeymoon without our three sons, all of whom were now in their late teens and busy with jobs, motor-cycles, and girlfriends. The boys saw us off with great relief and we drove to the French Riviera for a fortnight at Le Lavandou. We lazed on the beaches, made day excursions into St Tropez and Marseilles when we weren't swimming, and gorged ourselves on local food and wine in the evenings. It was in so many ways a second honeymoon, not least because nineteen years earlier, just after we were married, we had toured the south of France on a motor-cycle.

The main topic of conversation on this particular holiday was how to develop the freedom which was ours now that the children were coming of age. Jean wanted to commit herself to something outside the home and work full-time if possible but she lacked special skills; although she had been a secretary twenty years ago, she had forgotten her shorthand and typing. Today she was a creative and worldly person with a tremendous amount of potential but she had no idea how to realize it. My career was approaching its peak; I had been a journalist for nearly thirty years, spending the last ten years as home affairs corres-

3

pondent for the *Sunday Times*. I had also found some satisfaction as a writer, having completed my second book that winter which was due for publication within the month. Both Jean and I wanted to spend more time indulging our special interests. In my case this was to develop whatever writing skills I had and in Jean's it was to start a career. We wanted to be free to live and do as we pleased; we felt we were approaching a time when we could be more selfish about our own lives.

After we returned from our holiday, my book was published and we were delighted to find that it was well received. I secured a commission from Penguin almost immediately to write a third. Jean and I had decided to celebrate the achievement by adding a new wing to our house in Billericay, just outside London, something we had longed to do for years, giving us a much grander master bedroom and an additional living room to which we could escape when the boys brought their friends home. The wing took three months for completion and we welcomed the change. Whether the rooms were for our own indulgence or would boost the selling price of the house if we were to move was irrelevant; we merely felt we owed ourselves the luxury of an extension and decided to enjoy it while it was there.

One day, not long after moving into the new wing, we had finished reading the Sunday papers in bed when I noticed Jean put down the colour supplement and stare out of the window. She seemed unusually reflective and after a pause of a few minutes she said very simply, 'There's something worrying me, Derek.'

Because I knew that she was not one to suffer trifles, I was curious and asked her what the problem was. She replied that she had discovered a very small lump in her left breast the previous day. Because there was a history of cancer in her family, she had always been careful to examine herself for lumps in the breast as well as to have regular vaginal smears. Now she had found the tell-tale sign that every woman dreads. She asked me to examine her to confirm or allay her suspicions and when I did so there was no denying that at the crease below the breast, tucked close to the armpit, was a lump about the size of a pea.

We decided that she must see a doctor the next day and telephoned at once for an appointment early Monday morning. I could see that she was unsettled and I tried to soothe her by suggesting

4

that the lump could be any number of things although I was hard put to say exactly what. However, there were other ailments known to affect the breast and I emphasized this fact. To prevent her from brooding any longer, I got out of bed and she followed; we spent a pleasant Sunday without once alluding to her discovery. Jean consulted the family doctor the next morning and returned after a two hour absence looking bright and sanguine. 'He thinks it's mastitis,' she explained, 'and that with a bit of treatment it will go away.' She reiterated much of what the doctor had said, emphasizing that mastitis is a clot in the mammary system not at all uncommon in women of her age who have breast-fed their children. Certainly the diagnosis struck us as plausible and we were quite prepared to accept this possibility, feeling more than a little consoled by the explanation. However, tests and treatment were necessary to confirm the mastitis and arrangements had been made for Jean to visit the out-patient department of the Southend General Hospital the following week. The appointment was fixed for Monday afternoon, a convenient time for us since we were in the habit of driving to Southend weekly to do our shopping and treating ourselves to a long lunch and a ramble down the promenade. We finished our shopping early and had lunch before we reported to the hospital at three o'clock. Amongst other checks, some of the fluid from Jean's mammary system was drawn off and she was told to return a week later for the results of the tests.

If Jean was worried at all during that week she concealed it well and I had weathered too many years as a hard-nosed reporter to anticipate trouble before it hits you in the eye. However, it was evident to me when we did return to the hospital the following week that there was unmistakable tension beneath our placid composure. We both knew what we stood to lose if results confirmed that the lump was a malignant growth and not mastitis. Having known Jean for as long as I had, I could feel her apprehension distinctly. The waiting room was overflowing with patients so after we checked in at the main desk, we bought several magazines and settled down for a good read: we anticipated a lengthy wait. After what seemed like a long twenty minutes, Jean's name was called and she disappeared down the corridor leading to the consultants' offices. After just a moment on my own, I realized I was becoming fretful; wanting to escape the monotony of the waiting room, I decided to visit the canteen for a cup of tea. I willed myself to be optimistic but it required some effort. A sense of dread lingered over me which I could not altogether shrug off.

I finished my tea and returned to the waiting room where I tried to concentrate on observing the sea of faces in front of me. I had tried reading and found I could not pay attention and the time dragged on interminably. Eventually Jean appeared from one of the corridors, clutching a large brown envelope. Although she was quite a distance from me I could see her eyes fixed on mine as she approached. As she turned to place the documents on the receptionist's desk, I observed that her mouth was constricted and I knew this was not a good sign. When she sat down beside me I asked her immediately, 'How did it go?'

She looked away from me and there was a long silence. Then she said very quietly, 'He won't really tell me but there is a chance of cancer.'

We sat there absolutely dazed, trying to absorb the fact that a remote possibility had suddenly become a disquieting probability. I handed Jean her coat as I gathered up the magazines, and we began walking out of the hospital. I asked her what was going to happen now.

'I've got to come into hospital,' was all she said and I could sense by the finality in her tone that she didn't want to talk any more. We got into the car and drove the twenty miles back to Billericay in utter silence, each of us absorbed in our own thoughts. I wondered what was going to happen to her now and how she would cope with future problems as well as how much we should confide in the boys.

Once we had arrived home, Jean walked through the front door, sank into an armchair and burst into tears. I felt totally helpless and somewhat awkward knowing that the most I could do was sit on the edge of the chair with my arms around her as she continued to sob. For years Jean had spoken of the certainty that one day she would get cancer but she had reassured herself that it would happen when she was in her sixties and by then a cure would have been found. She had reason for her apprehension: her maternal grandmother, her own mother, and three of her aunts in this line had contracted cancer. The other two of six sisters died of heart attacks.

'Why has this happened to me so soon?' she cried bitterly. 'Why the hell have I developed it twenty years before the rest of my family?'

I tried taking a more positive line by asking what was going to happen now. She became calmer as she explained that she had to go to the hospital for an exploratory operation in which a tiny piece of the affected area is removed; while she was anaesthetized a pathologist would examine the tissue under a microscope. If the lump proved malignant the breast would then be removed. I took the opportunity to stress that the lump might still be non-cancerous, adding that even if it were not benign it had been detected early enough for treatment. Jean was strong and healthy and with good care would be able to fight it off. I consoled us both with this knowledge and observed that once again she put on a brave face and went into the kitchen to prepare dinner. After a few minutes I could hear her banging pots and pans and slamming cupboard doors, a sure sign that she was relieving tension and had survived this particular storm. A few minutes later our youngest son Stephen, who worked locally, arrived home and I left him chatting with Jean about his new job and slipped out of doors where I could be alone for a minute.

At the far end of the garden was a wooden shed where the boys kept their cycles and we kept our garden tools and furniture. I entered the shed and sat down on an old deck-chair, relieved to have a moment of solitude, for I needed to think things over on my own. During those few moments of seclusion, I could no longer deny to myself that things were serious; my previous optimism began to dissolve and I broke down. It took me about twenty minutes before I was able to regain my composure. I realize now when I emerged from the shed I had made my first acknowledgement that this was the beginning of the end. Yet curiously I was able simultaneously to pigeon-hole it in some recess of my mind, for I felt compelled to behave as if nothing unsettling had happened; in my more conscious thoughts, at any rate, I was determined to hope for the best and this somewhat lulled my own anxiety. The last thing I wanted to do was upset Jean so I left the shed and made a great show of waving to her as I passed the kitchen window

7

on my way to weed a flower-bed at the bottom of the garden.
That night during dinner we told the boys that their mother
would be going into the hospital for a small operation although
neither Jean nor I mentioned the possibility of cancer. It was less a
question of withholding information than the fact that we
simply were not certain ourselves. To have acknowledged the
possibility openly to the boys would have seemed a confirmation
of our worst fears and both Jean and I were adamant about
remaining hopeful. A few days later, a note arrived from the
hospital informing us that a bed had been reserved for Jean the
following week.

The promptness with which the hospital summoned Jean in-
sinuated the worst possible fears into her mind. To her, being so
hastily called for confirmed her worst misgivings. I pointed out
that it was only routine for the hospital to act so quickly and that
they did this in every case, emphasizing that we should concentrate
on enjoying the Christmas holidays rather than brood about
hypothetical problems. Thus we all made a concerted effort to
celebrate a quiet Christmas together, never once referring to the
impending operation which was in fact very much on our minds.
I knew that Jean was distressed but, typically, she showed
remarkable self-control and kept her apprehensions to herself.
When the scheduled day arrived, I drove Jean to Southend
and escorted her into the ward where she changed into night-
clothes and I arranged her things in a parcel to take home. She
was very stalwart about entering hospital, having been admitted
several times in the past for minor ailments, and she seemed
philosophical and cheerful. The operation was timed for later on
that afternoon so she suggested that I carry on with my own routine
and return that evening. We kissed good-bye and her parting words
to me were, 'Don't worry, I'll be all right.'
I drove the sixty miles to London where I had arranged to have
lunch with Commander Kenneth Newman, head of Scotland
Yard's Community Relations Department, who was later to
become Chief Constable of Northern Ireland. Our rendezvous was
a fashionable Italian seafood restaurant in the Strand. I arrived
somewhat late and, finding nowhere to park my car, abandoned

it outside the BBC in Bush House and hastened into the restaurant to find Newman waiting for me. Over lunch I told him of my plans to go to New York in order to interview their police chief and my intention of travelling further on to the West Indies to write about the political situation in the different islands. During the entire time I spoke with Newman I was preoccupied with thoughts of Jean and by the suspicion that I was a hypocrite for I knew there was a strong possibility that I would not be going abroad. However, things at that moment were too much in the balance to tell Newman and after a long lunch he wished me a good trip and I returned to my car which was smeared with parking tickets.

On the long drive back to the hospital I played the car radio in an effort to keep my mind off Jean, who was on the operating table about the time I started the drive out of London. I had been told by the Sister at the hospital not to telephone but to receive news of Jean that evening when I visited the ward. On the way to Southend I picked up our eldest son, Edgar, and arrived at the hospital just after six o'clock. We took the lift to the fifth floor and I asked Edgar to wait for me while I went into the Sister's office at the ward entrance. I entered the office and asked, 'How is she? Did you have to take the breast off?'

'She's fine,' the nurse replied, 'although still groggy. Yes, we had to remove the breast.'

The impact of the dreaded news made me feel wretched. I knew that this could be the beginning of a series of disasters. I wanted to see Jean immediately and I hurried towards her bed but before I reached it I realized I had not asked the nurse whether she knew the result of the operation. I had a sinking feeling that Jean did not know and I would have to tell her what had happened. I approached her bed in the corner of a pastel blue ward; beige curtains were drawn around her for she was not long out of the recovery room. As I stood at her bedside I could see that she was dozing so I sat down and just watched her for a while. After a few moments she stirred and I said softly, 'Hello love,' leaning over to kiss her. She was obviously very drugged and spent an instant gathering her thoughts. 'Did they take it off?' she asked drowsily.

I swallowed hard, knowing that there was no way I could

avoid levelling with her. 'Yes, they did, my darling,' I answered, whereupon she burst into convulsive sobs, unable to mumble anything coherent. A nurse heard her crying and came to give her an injection which had an immediate effect. The speed with which she lost consciousness unsettled me, frightened me really, for she became utterly inanimate within seconds and appeared to be dead. I sat beside the bed for a moment, quite numb from the awful news and Jean's emotional breakdown. I wondered what was to become of us in the months ahead.

Perhaps it was a feeling of overwhelming oppressiveness that made it difficult for me to move and it was with some effort that I staggered out of the ward; when I reached the corridor I started to cry. Edgar took hold of me, leading me to a corner by the elevator shaft where I sobbed on his shoulder like a small child. At that point he did not know the seriousness of Jean's illness but that made no difference to the quality of strength and comfort he gave me.

When I had managed to pull myself together we went out to the car and I let Edgar drive. As we edged towards Billericay, I told him all the details of the operation and explained all the possible consequences which he listened to with compassion and under-standing. I suggested that with the breast gone there was every chance that the cancer had been arrested in time and we must all look on the bright side of things. As I was working to console Edgar, offering the most hopeful prognosis, I realize now that I was working just as earnestly to convince myself as well. When we arrived at home, I explained the situation to the two other boys, who appeared stunned and baffled, and took the news silently apart from saying, 'Poor Mum.' To distract myself from fretting about Jean too much, I watched a third-rate movie on television that evening, made a cup of hot chocolate, and went to bed. It had been a taxing day and I soon fell asleep although I woke before dawn and lay in bed turning things over in my mind for several hours.

As soon as I arrived at the office the following morning I cancelled my trip to America and wrote to the Chief of the New York Police Department apologizing for the change in plans. The news editor, Del Mercer, suggested that I postpone the Caribbean trip for a month and see how things progressed when Jean came out of hospital. That evening I took Clive with me to see Jean and I was amazed at the dramatic change in her condition. She was sitting up in bed with the curtains drawn fully back and greeted us with a wide smile. Her face was pale but she was otherwise well and very cheery. I was heartened by this quick mental recovery although I realized that the euphoria was probably due in part to the effect of tranquillizers. After we kissed, the first thing that Jean did was ask about my trip to New York and emphasize that on no account was I to change my plans because of her. She was adamant about this so I replied as diplomatically as possible that of course I would carry on with my plans athough there would be a slight postponement. There was no question of my sacrificing the trip, I stressed; it had merely been delayed a few weeks and she readily accepted this compromise. Naturally she wanted to know how we were managing at home and I assured her that the boys and myself were eating heartily and coping well. We chatted quite gaily and the fact that she was a bit 'high' made things effortless for me; the visiting hour passed all too quickly. She made no reference to the loss of the breast except to say that she expected to leave the hospital in approximately ten days' time.

It was when I visited her the following evening that she was full of talk about the mastectomy. She pointed out a woman in the ward who had had a similar operation several years previously (she was now in the hospital for varicose veins) and mentioned other women she had been hearing about who had survived for scores of years after having had breasts removed. The hospital had sent a member of the staff to Jean's bedside earlier that day to discuss the breast replacement and Jean related to me all the alternative forms of 'prosthesis', a new word to me, which means an artificial replacement for parts of the body. She elaborated on the composition of different types of breast prosthesis – foam rubber, plastic, and cotton, to name several – and said that the National Health would provide two free of charge. If they proved unsatisfactory it was not too expensive to order one from a specialist surgical garment manufacturer.

Jean assured me that all the doctors were confident that the growth, even if it were malignant, had been caught in time and that we had nothing to fear. For the rest of her stay in the hospital

11

her spirits remained optimistic and if anyone had asked me if I thought I was going to lose her I would have replied most emphatically that it was unlikely. I began to put aside my scepticism and listened only to the hopeful stories of women who had had mastectomies and continued to live long and healthy lives. Any statistics on cancer which I came across I chose to interpret in a favourable way. Subconsciously I was filtering information and I became adept at developing perceptual gaps which precluded my hearing any unpromising figures.

With Jean's encouragement and blessing I made every effort to return to my hectic professional life. I told the office I would be ready to go to the West Indies in a month's time and I had no qualms about going. Jean left the hospital on schedule and kept herself occupied by dabbling in incidental household duties for we all encouraged her to take things easy for a while. The operation wound was covered with a massive Elastoplast bandage so I had not yet seen the scar. I knew Jean was sensitive about the loss of such an important part of her body; consequently whenever she referred to it I stressed how it made absolutely no difference to my feelings for her. I was just grateful that she was there and surviving. I noticed, however, that she now undressed with her back to me and never got into bed without a nightie on. When the bandage was removed three weeks later, she showed me – reluctantly – the long scar which was at least eight inches long and looked like a bright red weal, for the skin had not yet had a chance to grow. I tried to reassure her that it did not look too unsightly and that with time it would heal over. I was aware that I would get used to it gradually although I realized that nothing would ever compensate for the loss of so feminine a part of a woman's body. I went out of my way to comfort Jean by emphasizing how inconsequential it was in the light of the quality and durability of our love. I really meant it.

After a month her physical and emotional recovery seemed assured with the exception of a minor difficulty in raising her left arm above shoulder height. Her frame of mind and composure were excellent so I had no scruples about leaving her to go to the West Indies, knowing the boys would look after her well. She was returning to her old political and welfare activities and we seemed well on our way to resuming our normal life together.

3   ACTION THERAPY

When I returned from my month's tour of the West Indies I telephoned Jean from Heathrow Airport and was overjoyed to hear that she was so well, fit enough to offer to drive into central London to meet me. When we met outside Liverpool Street Station she pointed out – almost before saying hello – how embarrassed she was that one side of our Volvo was smashed in. She had been driving into a car park and while extracting a ticket from the automatic machine had let the car coast into a pillar. I told her not to worry, stressing that the important thing was that she was unhurt. The incident indicated two things to me above all: physically she was not able to handle a heavy car at slow speeds and perhaps her movement was handicapped in other ways as well, but psychologically she was coping admirably, almost normally, and it was this aspect I chose to concentrate on.

Two days after my return we drove to Bristol to celebrate my father's seventieth birthday. A six-week sabbatical holiday was due to me and Jean had agreed that it would be an ideal opportunity to write my next book. So we combined the birthday festivities with a search for a country cottage in nearby Somerset which would provide a creative environment. We had heard from a friend that a cottage not far from Bistol would be vacant that spring so we drove to the lovely cathedral town of Wells to view it. My

13

boyhood had been spent in the Mendip Hills just above Wells so I was keen to renew my connections. The cottage turned out to be ideal – quite small with timbered ceilings and an open fire – with just the right atmosphere for us both, so we contacted the owner immediately and made arrangements to rent it from mid-March to the end of April.

By now Jean was accepting the loss of the breast with little effort. Her personal embarrassment had dwindled and our love life had resumed normally. Occasionally she would allude to the absence of her breast, lamenting that she was less of a woman because of the operation but her complaints were short-lived. I invariably discouraged them for I could see no reason to indulge ourselves in regrets over things irrevocably gone; Jean's good health and spirits and mere presence were so vital to me that the scar and what it represented cosmetically were really unimportant. The strength of our marriage bond must have had a great deal to do with her equanimity as well. I came to see my role as diverting her attention away from the consequences of the operation in addition to providing testimony to the fact that love can be fortified through shared hardships. The boys were extremely understanding, agreeing with my philosophy, and it was reassuring to see Jean in the early morning wearing her housecoat without first putting on her prosthesis, not in the least minding that the boys could see the unevenness of her chest. She was accepting the mastectomy as a fact of life which had the same inevitability as the losing of one's wisdom teeth and within the family circle it did not matter to her who knew or what they thought. She began to accept that the insertion of the false breast was fundamentally no different from a woman applying make-up or wearing flattering clothes.

I could see a toughness emerging in Jean which interested me because I had always known it was there, a characteristic masked in part by her easy-going adaptable exterior, although up until now largely dormant. Her character had been formed in the 1930s during a childhood spent in the slums of Manchester when her father had been unable to find work for many years at a stretch. The family income was on a bare subsistence level and it was only through the shrewd house-keeping efforts and self-sacrifice of a conscientious mother that Jean was able to grow

14

into a tall and sturdy young woman with fair skin and flaxen hair. The harshness of the economic circumstances surrounding her in the depressive environment of Hulme brought out a desire to fight for something better and by the time she was sixteen she was working for the Communist Party as a leaflet distributor, becoming a member of the Young Communist League the following year. This was after 1945, the time of the West's honeymoon with Russia, when food was rationed and social conditions were bleak. For all the ordinary person knew, Britain was going to resume the pre-war pattern of massive dole queues and widespread deprivation yet again.

By 1950 Jean had left the Communists and joined the Labour League of Youth in a newly-built subsidized housing development on the outskirts of Manchester to which her family had moved. When the fledgling district (Wythenshawe) organized its first carnival it ran a contest to find the young person who best represented the 'flower of young womanhood' to be their carnival queen. Egged on by her father, Jean entered herself as a candidate. The first year she was runner-up; the second year she won, more for her poise, personality, and the punch of her little speech than for her good looks, as she never considered herself a glamorous woman. She carved a small niche in local history as the first 'political' Miss Wythenshawe and she held office for a year, making the round of charities, balls, and hospitals. She worked hardest at the civic duties during her reign, for she saw her role in life as a campaigner for political change. She continued to crusade for the Labour Party during the 1950 and 1951 elections during which time she became unpopular with older members of the party for a speech in which she castigated them for spending too much time drinking in the Labour Club and not enough time vote-gathering.

She directed all her energies into organizing youth club activities and it was when she became chairman of the Wythenshawe Youth Council that I interviewed her as a young reporter working in the district for the *Manchester Evening News*. I fell in love with her at that interview and very much wanted to date her. Despite my training in aggressiveness as a journalist, I was painfully shy in other respects and shrank at the idea of telephoning or confronting Jean directly. However, it occurred to me to buy two

15

tickets to a Hallé Concert at the Free Trade Hall and write her a letter thanking her for the interview, adding a postscript that I had some spare concert seats and had enclosed one ticket if she cared to use it. Congratulating myself on my resourcefulness, I took my seat on the night of the concert well before the warming-up overture only to endure the anguish of last-minute panic over the possibility that there would be an empty seat next to me all evening. However, Jean appeared as the house lights began to dim and our love affair started. Three weeks later we decided to get married and three weeks after that the little ceremony took place in the Manchester Registry Office at the Town Hall. Only our parents were invited. All other friends and relatives were stunned at the speed of our courtship but we were oblivious to public opinion and hopped onto my motor-cycle to spend our honeymoon touring the south of France, living in a tent and sleeping bags which we kept stowed in the cycle's side-panniers.

When we returned to Manchester we decided to start a family right away and had two sons within three years. Although Jean could easily have had more children, we adopted a third son four years after the birth of our youngest child. It came about when, in 1957, we were living in a suburban semi-detached house in south Manchester surrounded by neighbours whose lives seemed totally devoted to self-indulgent whims. Several had remarked to us over the garden fence that they were not going to have larger families because they wanted a new kitchen, a bigger car, or a new washing machine: all part of the keeping-up-with-the-Joneses syndrome. Our two boys were wonderfully healthy and well-cared for and it was around that time that I wrote several articles for my news-paper about the huge number of children living in Manchester's orphanages and foster homes, stressing how so few people wanted to adopt them, particularly those over two years old or with a racially-mixed background. I was talking with Jean one evening about the subject and to my astonishment she said, 'Well, I think we should adopt one. What's the good of bringing more and more children into the world while those crowded into orphanages are being dragged up?'

We considered the possibility for several weeks and then made a written application to the Manchester Corporation Children's Department who promptly sent a case worker to see us. At the end of the interview we were asked if we would be willing to take a child of any colour and we said that race did not matter so long as it was a boy of about three; we felt that this would be the most compatible arrangement with our own boys, now four and six. Shortly after that a charming lad called Stephen started to visit us on weekends and later for week-long periods. At the end of six months' permanent residence we formally adopted him. The illegitimate son of a half-African mother and white father, he had so far spent two of his three years in foster homes because his mother could not cope on her own with the stresses of family life. Stephen had blond kinky hair and the striking good looks often found in racially-mixed children. We felt our family was now complete with three robust sons and we looked forward to a world of possibilities to discover together.

Much as she wanted to, Jean refused to take any kind of employment while the boys were still at school. She continued to believe that a mother should be present when the children came home from school and be able to care for a child during any sickness without the outside pressures of having to go to work. Her attitude sprang from observing the multitude of 'latchkey children' surrounding her in the Manchester slums of her youth in the 1930s – children sent to school with the front door key attached to a piece of string around their necks – an inevitability when most mothers had little choice but to go to work or see the family slowly starve. To compensate for being at home so much, Jean took up political and welfare work. In addition to her active campaigning for the Labour Party, she served as a governor in three local schools, managed an Oxfam shop in Billericay, and helped with the hospital's book-lending service for patients – activities which she felt kept her in touch with other people, particularly those who could not always help themselves. In this way she felt she established an agreeable balance between providing the children with the attention they deserved and getting stimulation from outside the home which would prevent her from developing, in her eyes, a stodgy and domestically-bound mentality.

When the time came for my sabbatical holiday Jean and I drove out of London in two cars, my Volvo and her Daf, each filled to the brim with a small desk, typewriters, boxes of documents as well as our personal effects for a six-week stay. At the first rest station on the motorway, we stopped for coffee and Jean asked if we could change cars. With the restricted movement of her left arm, the tiny Daf had been suitable for edging through London's traffic but on the open road she wanted the more comfortable car. I set off in the sedate little Daf while Jean powdered her nose in the Ladies' Room but before I had travelled ten miles I noticed a Volvo just like ours screaming past me at something approaching one hundred miles an hour, disappearing over the brow of the hill. I caught a glimpse of Jean at the wheel as she flew by and I was struck by her sense of abandon. The impact of her vitality was a good indication of her powers of restitution.

At this point we were both eager for a change from Billericay and the grim associations it had recently held for us, so the rustic cottage provided a refreshing break. Here we were cramped, we kept hitting our heads on the ceiling beams, the log fire needed constant tending, and climbing the steep, winding staircase was an athletic feat, but we adored every minute of the inconvenience.

It was late March and the weather ranged from sharply cold with light snowfalls to pleasantly warm when the spring sunshine came up over the Mendip Hills. We arranged a work routine which consisted of my writing every morning from nine o'clock to one o'clock, followed by an afternoon of roaming the countryside. We would return to the cottage at dusk for our dinner, light the log fire, and spend the evening peacefully, with Jean reading and myself preparing for the next day's writing session. We were thankful not to have television; instead we listened to radio concerts or played our favourite music on a stereo tape machine. We walked a great deal during our afternoon excursions and Jean was fit enough to climb the Glastonbury Tor, a very steep hill. She looked in the bloom of health and as ever provided the calm, stable background so necessary for a writer. Conditions were so auspicious that I could see that it would be easy to complete the book within the six weeks of sabbatical leave which, in fact, I was able to do.

It was in late March, on Easter Saturday, that we made a spontaneous decision which was to change our lives dramatically. On the spur of the moment we decided to drive from Wells to

18

Chippenham, a distance of about twenty-five miles, to see two friends whom I had known when, after coming out of the army, I worked as a junior reporter for the *Bristol Evening World* covering the county of Wiltshire. My base was Chippenham and as a young bachelor I frequented the old coaching inn in the Market Place, the Angel, where I met the only two bohemian people in the area. They were known as Ricky and Bobby: in 'straight' life they were Mr Richardson, teacher of mathematics at the local grammar school, and Mrs Richardson, a former ballet dancer and art historian. It was their hobby to unofficially adopt bright young men and women in their twenties who were fretting over artistic failures or unrealized ambitions. Bobby and Ricky would inject a dose of self-confidence through imaginative suggestions, lots of conversation, and an abundance of booze. I was one of the many youngsters whose ambitions were given a necessary boost by their stimulating company during the 1950s and 1960s. They were not a shattering success in their own lives, but they had made peace with themselves, and enjoyed the uncanny knack of convincing their protégés that they – the younger ones – were those who would make it to the top.

Jean had met them only once ten years earlier but was as keen to see them as I was. We drove to their house in Kington Langley, a Cotswold village just outside Chippenham, only to find the garden gate locked and no means of communicating with anyone inside. Crossing a field to get around the back, Jean and I scaled the rear garden fence and started across the huge lawn towards the house, eventually confronting an astonished Bobby peering at us from a window. After her shock had subsided and recognition of us registered,she ran out to greet us crying, 'Well, I'll be buggered! Look who's turned up after all these years!' Ricky joined us and we went inside and lay on the floor for drinks – they did not approve of chairs– and began bringing one another up to date on our lives over the last ten years. Bobby asked if we were thinking of moving back to the West Country; I had been born in Bath only fourteen miles away and, like many people in their forties, I often felt the urge to return to my roots. I told her that we had considered the idea but we were not certain we could afford it yet because my career obviously lay with the *Sunday Times* for some time to come. Since arriving in Somerset, Jean and I had occasionally remarked to one another how pleasant it would be to live there but we had not gone so far as to make any concrete suggestions about moving.

Typically, Bobby seized on what was little more than a whim to tell us that an interesting old place – called Pinchloafe House – was for sale in the next village. A little shop went with the property. As soon as the word 'shop' was mentioned I could see Jean's eyes light up, so I asked for more details. Bobby promptly produced the real estate leaflet relating the specifications of the property. The house was priced at £28,000 but Bobby said that it could be bought for a good deal less because the owners were having trouble selling and were anxious to leave for business reasons. We considered the situation carefully and Bobby, typically the opportunist, instantly telephoned a mortgage broker so that he and I might discuss finances. While I was speaking with him, Jean asked lots of questions about the shop and learned that it was considerably run down but had potential for making money on a small scale.

We telephoned the owners for an appointment and were delighted when they suggested that we come right away. Within two hours of scaling Bobby and Ricky's wall we were viewing a house for sale. As we arrived in the tiny village of Langley Burrell, we were immediately struck with the beauty of Pinchloafe House. It was a Cotswold stone farmhouse, built in 1734, with a stone-tiled roof and mullion windows. There was a large front garden with an attached cottage; on the other side of the farmhouse was an addition constructed from newer Cotswold stone which was in fact the village shop. Adjacent to this were no less than eight garages. At the rear of the house there was a long garden with a small orchard. The inside of the farmhouse had been modernized a bit too brashly for our liking but on the whole it was in excellent condition and would require no renovation. The ground floor seemed to sprawl in several directions: it included a breakfast room with a well-worn, stone-slabbed floor adjacent to a modern kitchen with adjoining conservatory, a large square living room (it had been the shop before the addition was built), and a dining room with extensive views of the front and rear gardens. On the first floor were three double bedrooms; the second storey attic was strikingly timbered and, although in need of restoration, provided what we felt was an exciting possibility for more bedrooms and a studio. The trade in the shop was, as we had been warned, so badly run down that virtually no accounts were kept but I could see Jean's eager response in sensing the challenge of improving the business. We thanked the owners for showing us their home and drove back to Bobby and Ricky's house. On our way to Kington Langley Jean remarked with unconcealed enthusiasm, 'I could certainly make something of that shop and it would give me plenty to do.'

This comment really finalized my decision to put an offer in to buy Pinchloafe House. I had been initially struck by the fact that it was the kind of home I had always dreamed of and now, with Jean's obvious attraction to it, I realized that if it were at all possible I was going to purchase the house for us both. What had impressed me more than anything else in the past few weeks was how a change in environment had produced such a radical improvement in Jean's spirits. She was happier away from Billericay where well-meaning people kept providing unwelcome reminders of her illness by asking how she was and what the medical prognosis was for the future. I sensed that the old maxim about a 'clean break' was valid in our circumstances and would bring Jean a great deal of happiness for whatever time remained to her.

For years we had both dreamed of living in the country and – in being painfully honest with myself – I now had to consider the likelihood of Jean not reaching old age. This was undoubtedly the moment to act. Not least important was the fact that the shop would provide the right kind of vocation for her now that our sons were about to start their own adult lives. Without a family to care for, the ever-present fear of the cancer returning could insinuate itself into Jean's mind and so easily agitate her unless she had some kind of healthy preoccupation. The fact that we knew nothing about keeping a shop did not daunt us; on the contrary, it would demand all of Jean's attention as well as prove a valuable experience. The *Sunday Times* could continue to provide our main income although the move would mean that I would have to live alone in London four days a week. However, what stood out in my mind was the realization that were Jean to become seriously ill we would be near enough to my family, most of whom lived in

21

Somerset or Dorset, to appeal to them for help if necessary. I admitted to myself that the whole thing might not be the wisest financial endeavour but, on the whole, there were so many advantages for Jean. This fact took top priority in my mind.

When we returned to Kington Langley we told Bobby that we wanted the house so long as it could be bought for not more than £22,000 and, being fairly skilled in real estate negotiation, she offered to act as our representative. We would not know for several hours if our offer was acceptable so Jean and I decided to drive to Bath for dinner and telephone Bobby at eight o'clock that evening for news. At the end of a long meal in a local inn during which there had been only one topic of conversation, I hurried to phone Bobby to find out what had happened. After an ecstatically short conversation, I ran back to tell Jean, 'It's ours for £20,000!' For a moment we were both too incredulous to speak. Jean was overwhelmed, as was I, at the thought of owning an old Cotswold farmhouse, a shop, a cottage, and eight garages. We were as eager as two adolescents over our new acquisition and I relished the prospect of living in the country again for the first time since I was fifteen. We laughed over the fact that we had set out at eleven o'clock that morning merely to call on old friends and by eight o'clock were the owners of an impressive country home a hundred miles away from our suburban London house.

My sabbatical ended four weeks later and Jean and I returned to London to tell relatives and friends that not only were we moving house but setting up shop as well. Needless to say, everyone was astounded because they had had no idea we ever intended moving – although admittedly neither had we until that Easter Saturday. The owners of Pinchloafe House had stipulated that they would sell us the farmhouse, cottage and shop at the lower price of £20,000 only if the deal were completed within six weeks so I had to hustle to sell our Billericay home in order to get sufficient funds to make the move. I put the property in the hands of several local agents and waited for a stream of callers, only to discover that very few came. I was unaware that the boom in the housing market had suddenly ended. From a position where people had been buying houses during 1971 and 1972, occasionally without even seeing the property before bidding because competition was so fierce, now the same type of house could sit for months without attracting any potential buyers despite falling prices. However, we continued to be hopeful although we realized that it might take longer to sell than we had hoped.

As we made concrete plans to change our way of life so radically, I noticed how Jean's philosophy of life was changing too. She had never been one to suffer fools or hypocrites gladly and she could be quite brusque with anyone whom she considered insincere or selfish. However, she now showed more tolerance towards others and she would often say, 'There's simply no point in attacking anyone.' Her attitude towards her own health and future became more calculating and she pointed out to me more than once, 'I know that I might live only four or five years more and so I'm going to live, live, live!' This was an altogether new kind of self-indulgence. I could see how she wanted to shrug off our London life and all its drab assocations, live in the country in a rustic old farmhouse and, most of all, run that shop. I felt able to take chances because I had proved my ability to sell books and articles as well as appearing on the occasional radio and television programme, all of which supplemented my income from the newspaper. I readily fell in with Jean's philosophy of getting the best out of life; it was such a happy sign that she was taking the initiative in developing a vivacious and outgoing manner that I was quite prepared to give every support.

Within a fortnight of returning from Wells, Jean was due back at the hospital for a routine check-up. Neither of us was in the least worried as we drove to Southend. It was a glorious spring day as I delivered Jean to the out-patient's department and I sat basking in the sun on the lawn in front of the hospital waiting for her to return. A half-hour later she came up behind me and joined me on the grass. I was so unsuspecting of trouble that I was not looking at her closely when she stated, 'I've got to come back into hospital again for another operation. They've got to remove the lymph glands.' I could see that she was crest-fallen and I felt myself fighting off the edge of panic when I considered the implications of this latest medical bulletin. We walked to the car and drove home in no mood to take our stroll along the sea front as we had intended. We did not talk during the drive to Billericay and I could see that Jean was deep in her thoughts as was I. For the entire thirty minute journey I tried to weigh up the options for handling this new crisis.

By the time we arrived home the tension erupted. We collapsed in one another's arms on the sofa, spilling out our misery by weeping bitterly. The ominous news destroyed the euphoria we had felt over her remarkable recovery as well as our impending move to Wiltshire. It was Jean who declared, 'We're *not* moving, we're not going down to Chippenham.' I had not expected this extreme reaction and to play for time I told her we must think about the situation carefully. She sensed then, as did I, that the cancer had travelled too extensively in her body to be mastered by surgery, drugs, or X rays.

'I'm not even going to live as long as I thought,' she cried bitterly. 'We're not going to move house because I've got a lot less time and I can't burden you with my illness and coping with a house and shop.'

My overwhelming intuition was that an unqualified surrender to this setback – which would mean cancelling the move to Wiltshire – would end all hope. Preventing any further hesitation, I said very strongly, 'We *are* moving. We're going to Wiltshire – we've made a deal and we're going through with it.' Without replying, Jean got up from the sofa and went into the kitchen to put the kettle on for a cup of tea. A few minutes later she came back into the living room, looked me straight in the eye and declared, 'All right. Let's go there and by all means let's live the best and fullest life possible regardless of what lies ahead.'

I adored her for her courage and self-possession. From this moment on she developed a strategy of positive thinking from which she never wavered despite the operation, painful X-ray treatment, and considerable difficulties in trying to sell the London house. 'I really am going to make the most of my life,' Jean said later on, more than once. 'I'm going to live high.' Such remarks were made to fortify her own morale yet, so far as I could see, she had every intention of realizing them. In order to cope with the horror of her situation she had turned away from thinking about the long-term future and had adopted a philosophy of seizing the immediate moment – the *carpe diem* which poets lyricize about – which often bordered on a devil-may-care extreme. About a week

24

after our decision to continue with our plans, Jean was driving her little Daf to the shopping centre in Basildon and had to stop on a hill behind a long queue of traffic. A lorry approaching from behind failed to brake in time and hit Jean's car with such a thrust that it concertina-ed the Daf between the lorry and the vehicle in front of Jean, folding in both front and rear ends of the car. Yet she kicked her way out of the door, telephoned a taxi and arrived home quite unaffected. Apart from acknowledging her good fortune in not being hurt. she was not in the least mentally shaken. 'Poor old car!' was all she said – and she jumped in the Volvo setting off, once again, on her shopping expedition.

Her self-control remained intact and when the day came for the second operation Jean was in excellent spirits. The removal of the glands was a relatively simple procedure, involving an operation just behind the armpit. Hospitalization would not be too extensive and Jean hoped that she would be able to leave after a week or ten days if all went well. Some doctors consider it part of their normal routine to remove the lymph glands at the same time that the mastectomy is performed, making the operation slightly more extensive. However, just as frequently, doctors prefer to perform a less radical mastectomy, leaving the glands intact until further evidence indicates that removal is necessary. This was so in Jean's case; tests had shown the lymph glands to be active with cancer and the operation was performed as quickly as possible followed by radio-therapy treatment.

Despite the discomfort caused by X-ray burns to the skin, Jean helped us prepare for the move by packing endless parcels and cartons. However, she could not accompany us on the move because she had several more radio-therapy sessions scheduled at the hospital. Edgar and Clive had decided to move to Wiltshire with us and I appreciated their help and presence, for Jean would need the company while I was working in London. Stephen was feeling restless at home and was deeply troubled over questions of his adoption and racial identity so that when he said he preferred to remain in London we all agreed that this was best. He had found lodgings with a West Indian family and it was a necessary broadening of his experience to live with a black family in a multiracial, working-class district after an upbringing in an all white, middle-class area. At school he had been tormented by other

25

students about being a 'half-caste' and was dubbed 'Rastus'. 'What am I, black or white?' he would ask us desperately. 'You're just a human being,' Jean would say.

Jean's father had lived alone in Manchester since his wife's death from lung cancer in 1967 so Jean pressed him to join us in Wiltshire. She wanted his help in the shop as well as his company when I was at work in London. He agreed to come although he was not keen to leave his roots and friends. However, he realized that his only daughter might not have long to live so he made his arrangements to move to Wiltshire. When we left Billericay there was still no buyer in sight for the house and I was obliged to take a bridging loan from the bank in order to purchase the Chippenham property. To provide cash to stock the shop we sold Jean's car. Thus when the boys and I followed the removal van to Langley Burrell we had firm instructions from Jean that the shop was to be closed for one week only and that she would be there at the end of her treatment to re-open it in style.

Pinchloafe House looked far less picturesque when we arrived at the end of June, for it had been a wet spring and the previous owners had let the garden deteriorate into utter anarchy. Nettles in the orchard loomed as high as five feet and the rose bushes drooped over the paths to such an extent that I had to hack away the prickly runners before the furniture men could approach the house. It took us two days to unpack and we then had to set about the awesome task of stocking the shop. Clive and I scrubbed it down, clearing away the reams of toilet paper and vast quantities of baby food which had been left behind. We then drove twenty miles to a wholesale cash-and-carry grocers in Swindon to begin the re-stocking.

As I walked down the avenues of food and dry goods piled high in the enormous warehouse it became apparent to me that I had absolutely no idea what I was doing. What *did* the typical English store sell? I realized that the only answer was to see the problem in terms of what *I* would need on a shopping expedition of my own so I started with biscuits, jam, marmalade, tinned fruit, shoe polish, tinned vegetables, cereal, and soap. When I completed the inventory, I loaded the contents into my car and drove back to the shop where Clive and I began to lay out the shelves. As we were doing this, we realized the scores of items which we had missed. Making a note of each of these, we returned to the wholesalers the following day to fill in the many gaps. Several trips were required and this was a tedious process, but by Saturday when Jean arrived by train, the shop looked abundantly replenished and she was well pleased with our efforts. Now at full tilt, she spent the weekend adjusting shelf and window displays and pricing all the goods.

When I told the boys that the second operation seemed to have been entirely successful and that the possibility of cancer had passed, I hinted to them -- although they hardly needed it -- that the subject of their mother's health was now closed. We were not going to tell anyone in Wiltshire what had happened; I stressed how this was to be a totally fresh start for us all. Because they had dreaded discussing Jean's illness in the past, my suggestion was welcomed by them. With so much to occupy us in our new home and the novelty of the shop, Jean and I easily reverted to our old optimism and we were happy to let the future take care of itself. The shop was to be the vital therapy for Jean and, with her strong body and healthy good looks, the prospects were encouraging.

Despite our reticence about Jean's illness, some of the side-effects did not escape a keen and inquiring eye. A neighbour appeared unexpectedly while Jean was stacking shelves in the shop and unknown to her her blouse was slightly open at the cleavage, revealing a tell-tale indelible ink mark made by the radiographers with which to guide the path of the X ray. 'What's that blue mark on your skin?' the woman asked, quick as a flash. 'It's some treatment I've been having,' Jean replied, instantly dismissing the subject. However, she was left with the distinct feeling that this woman understood the reason for the mark and that the news would soon make the rounds of the village gossips. There was nothing we could do about it so we chose to ignore the matter. There was simply too much to look forward to with our new responsibilities and emerging life-style.

4 GOOD TIMES

Jean needed no alarm clock to alert her on Monday morning and she got up well in time to launch her shop at 9 A.M. She put on a smart red pinafore and unbolted the doors at 8.45. I painted the words 'Shop Open Today' on a large board and nailed it to the fir tree at the entrance to the gate. Our first customer was the elderly village squire, Major Ash, whom we had been eagerly expecting, for other villagers had advised us that he would make it a point of principle to be the first customer in order to demonstrate his support for local trade. He drove up in a battered old Vauxhall and marched in clutching a tiny slip of paper which contained a list of shopping items. He lived alone and needed few provisions. The bucolic old gentleman in his oversized trousers and rubber boots imperiously informed us about his preferences from which he claimed he never deviated. 'I only buy ginger marmalade, you know, and I only smoke that particular kind of tobacco,' he snorted, pointing to his private tobacco pouch. 'Kindly make certain that you stock all these things.' Jean and I took copious notes while assuring him that we would make every effort to provide him with whatever he preferred.

As other customers began to file into the shop, Jean and I worked out a routine whereby she did the actual selling while I made note of the many items we were short of and by the end of the day, with a fairly brisk trade, we had a very long list indeed.

29

Practically all the village ladies had made an appearance, no doubt motivated less by a desire to buy than to assess us as the new resident shopkeepers of Langley Burrell but they all made a concerted effort to wish us well. Like the squire, most of our customers proclaimed loud and clear exactly what they would like to see in stock. Soon Jean and I began to realize that what everyone craved was an exclusive, personal service catering to their every whim. If we bought a crate of a desired item and sold it at the rate of one a week to suit the one person who had wished to see it stocked, we were going to need an enormous amount of capital.

For the first week the shop did an exceptionally lively trade. Everyone continued to come in and take a look around and offer encouragement. Although she was a city girl, Jean loved talking to the customers and she soon became very much 'persona grata' with the villagers. They were friendly and well-meaning and always bought something although the amount spent was often nominal. We decided that it was best to close the shop on Tuesdays in order to visit the warehouse to replenish our stock. We would stay open from 9 A.M. to 6 P.M. on other weekdays, hoping that the longer hours of business would provide us with some kind of profit.

Not long after we opened, I had to climb on the roof on a Tuesday afternoon to clean the storm gutters. As I was aloft I could see the village women with their shopping bags walking towards Chippenham, a two-mile trek. An hour later they returned with their bags fully laden, indicating to me that the women did their main shopping in the town's supermarkets and used our shop for the odds and ends which they had forgotten or run short of. I neglected to mention this observation to Jean because I did not want to dampen her enthusiasm. Having been reared in the West Country I knew that these hardy women enjoyed the good walk to town and did not mind in the least humping the heavy packages home.

The shop had a refreshing, clean appearance with good lighting and smart, open shelving. Jean displayed the goods with a real flair for style, making the shop appear better stocked than it actually was. Three deep freezes provided frozen vegetables, meat, and ice cream. We sold everything from potatoes to birthday cards and, despite my roof-top observations, trade appeared brisk even if the volume of goods sold was low. Quite a few of the villagers patronized us because they realized that without their trade the only shop in the village would disappear, as had happened once already. Our most frequent customers were the children who by no stretch of the imagination were big spenders. If flush, they would invest in twenty-five or fifty pence worth of goods but the usual amount was more like five or ten pence.

Three weeks after our move to Wiltshire we were so utterly absorbed in our new life we had forgotten about the cancer. Jean was becoming a competent organizer and could easily cope with the shop on her own so I made arrangements to return to London for my four-day working week. I rented a room from a friend in Clapham Junction and planned a divided existence commuting between London and Langley Burrell. Just before I returned to work, there occurred the only incident in which Jean alluded to her mastectomy. I had been decorating the farmhouse bathroom and had hung a large plate glass mirror there. Looking at it, she asked me to take it down. 'I don't really want it there, where I can see my operation scar every time I get out of the bath.' I decided it would be bad for her psychologically if I accepted her argument and I emphasized that this was the best possible place for the mirror adding that, by now, she ought to have accepted the scar. After all, I stressed, I had. It only needed this bit of prodding and firmness for her to acquiesce and she never once made another reference after that day to the lost breast.

Jean was anxious to get more involved in village affairs and when she was approached by the Women's Institute about becoming a member she felt she could not refuse. She did not relish this type of organization, preferring something more politically or socially orientated, but there was little alternative given our need for the goodwill of the village and increased patronage of the shop. She soon began to enjoy the Wednesday evening meetings and the other members, mostly farmers' wives, liked her frank and friendly manner. We both joined the local Labour Party, increasing its active membership from three to five. To reach their meeting-place we tramped across a field to a seventeenth-century stone cottage where we sat in a tiny parlour with a roaring log fire while the three party officials – chairman, secretary, and treasurer – conducted the business. Jean and I were the only 'plain' members.

Because we were 'tradespeople', and I was a professional journalist as well, we were accepted into another stratum of village society, that of the influential and well-to-do. Although we did not attend church, we were often invited to sherry parties given after the Sunday morning service by the vicar or squire or other local worthies. The level of conversation at these social gatherings was not, I noted, particularly elevating. One Tory lady, on being told that I worked for the *Sunday Times*, said gushingly, 'Then you must be terribly left wing!' 'Yes, I am,' I answered, more intent on shocking her than being truthful, until I realized as the conversation droned on that merely being in the Labour Party was considered radical. In referring to the awful 'left wing', she did not have in mind the far left International Socialists or International Marxist Group: merely being middle class and non-Tory meant that I was an aberration in her eyes. Nevertheless, Jean and I were to straddle the two layers of village society quite comfortably because of our joint occupations as journalist and shop-keeper as well as our membership in the Labour Party and Women's Institute. We cultivated our friendships on both levels by adhering to the two essential manners of country life which I had learned as a boy on a Somerset farm: never speak ill of your neighbour and always greet everyone you pass whether you know them or not. Jean campaigned on her own, going to garden fêtes, church hall bazaars and jumble sales, revelling in her new environment and her role as 'the lady who keeps the village shop'.

As we became more adept at stocking the shop we made fewer trips to the warehouse in Swindon and were able to spend our Tuesdays pursuing a recreation that developed into a mild addiction for us both. Because our farmhouse was so large we realized right away that it would require a great deal more furniture of a far older vintage than those pieces we had brought from London. We began to attend country auctions in nearby farmhouses or at salerooms in Bath and it became our habit to combine a visit to a sale with an interesting pub lunch. Within a few months we could see that the shop was a commercial disaster so we cheered ourselves up by going to more and more auctions. In fact, Jean was able to draw no salary at all despite her long hours of vigilance and the insurance, rates, and the shop's share of the mortgage more than swallowed its tiny profit. However, with her growing interest in antiques and the countryside, Jean began to make plans for another type of shop which would specialize in goods such as crafts or furniture reflecting different aspects of our Wiltshire surroundings. In the meantime we consoled ourselves with the knowledge that the majority of our own food came from the shop at wholesale prices. 'It's not so bad,' Jean would joke, 'we're eating our profits, literally!'

That autumn our eldest son, Edgar, although only eighteen, decided to get married. Curiously, Vivienne, with whom he was in love, was the great-granddaughter of Ernest and Kate Winter, a wonderful couple with whom I had lived as a boy evacuee on the Mendip Hills during the 1939-45 war. Our arguments that they should wait until they were older did not impress them and in early December they were quietly married at the Chippenham Town Hall. A few days later we celebrated their wedding with a big family party at Pinchloafe House which combined our house-warming and their reception, and the young couple moved into the adjacent Pinchloafe Cottage. We continued our festive mood by planning what we hoped would be a memorable Christmas day: in addition to our three sons, our new daughter-in-law and Jean's father, we invited my Aunt Gwen from Bristol, Godson Anosike, an eighteen-year-old refugee from the Biafran civil war, and Irvine Worland, a twenty-year-old West Indian poet to join us at Pinchloafe House. Although Jean's health seemed perfect, I wanted to protect her from any strain so I arranged that we should all go to a hotel in Bath for Christmas dinner. She was overjoyed that all the youngsters could join us, especially Godson and Irvine who had become like adopted sons. It was a radical change on her part to wish to celebrate Christmas in a flamboyant manner. Her high-spirited gaiety at the hotel contributed a great deal to everyone's hilarity. The festivities were carried on at home and at one point everyone donned paper hats and sang. We all remarked on what a joyful day it had been, attributing most of its success to Jean's infectious good cheer.

33

In January we took the shop's cash books to our accountant and asked him for a rapid assessment of any commercial progress and its prospects for the future. While we waited for his verdict, Jean related her intentions of either opening a craft shop or even transforming the house into a small private hotel during the summer season. This was her latest brainchild and in many ways not a bad idea: she felt that the long hours of keeping a shop were too constraining and offered too little reward financially and personally. With a private hotel, she would be able to convert the shop into a little flat for ourselves and put the paying guests into the timbered 'olde worlde' bedrooms in the main part of the farmhouse.

After perusing the records our accountant advised us that the shop had absolutely no prospect of making money and that I was heavily subsidising it from my own income, something I was altogether aware of without any confirmation from him. In addition to the liability of the shop as a commercial endeavour, we had still not sold our house in London despite its having been on the market for nine months and the interest on the bridging loan was mounting at an alarming rate. When we returned to Langley Burrell, Jean immediately announced to the village that, due to a shortage of customers and trade, the shop would close at the end of January. She was disappointed but not entirely surprised by its failure and during the last week of January she ran a closing-down sale disposing of the bulk of goods through slashed prices. Most of what was left we were able to consume in the months that followed. Villagers accepted the shop's closing stoically, several hinting that they had expected it, although there was widespread disappointment over the loss of a useful service. Not one to grieve over failure, Jean confirmed to me that she would like to press on with her plans for a private hotel and she began to buy an abundance of linen and blankets as well as several new beds so that she might open in the late spring. She drew up an advertisement centred around the attractions of the handsome old farmhouse in the rolling Wiltshire countryside and directed all her energies towards yet another major endeavour.

In the meantime we dabbled in trivial diversions enjoying our surplus of leisure time. The garden needed a good deal of work and at Jean's behest we enrolled in an evening class for gardeners at Lackham College of Agriculture, dutifully appearing

34

with notebooks and pens at the first Monday evening class. The subject of the lesson was an impressive lecture on how to grow orchids and Jean and I listened first in awe, then in embarrassment, and then in stupified boredom. The discussion was far too erudite for our amateur minds and I noticed with a sinking feeling that everyone else in the class was riveted to their seats. These country people had a far more thorough grounding in the art of gardening than either Jean or I had. On the following Monday afternoon we peered timidly at the programme and when we saw that the entire lecture was devoted to the growing of broad beans, we exchanged glum glances. I suggested, 'Should we go out to dinner somewhere instead?' and without a second's hesitation Jean nodded enthusiastic assent and we were off.

With the shop closed, Jean was also able to resume interest in what was to her a very serious activity – the world of politics. A general election was coming and she threw herself into work. The Chippenham Constituency Labour Party appointed her as deputy agent, a full-time and unpaid job which involved a heavy work-load and a great deal of responsibility. Despite the fact that the legal duties for conducting the election properly belonged to the main agent, he could not get release from his employment and Jean willingly assumed all the donkey work. When I visited her in the election headquarters I was agreeably surprised to see her in full command of the entire Labour campaign and it was with some difficulty that I managed to coax her away from her duties to have a pub lunch with me.

However, just as Jean was beginning to revel in the progress of her work effort, she experienced an unsettling bout of what appeared to be 'flu. I had driven to Birmingham to gather material for a political article and Jean and Vivienne decided to take a walk across the fields near home to a bird sanctuary. Conditions were worse than they expected and they had to wade along muddy tracks and tramp through long, dank grass; after an hour Jean's back began to ache badly and she became weak and ill. Vivienne had the greatest difficulty in getting her home – a distance of about a mile – and when they finally arrived back Jean went straight to bed for several days. The doctor diagnosed a bad attack of influenza which she had probably caught from Vivienne who had just recovered from it. Within a week Jean was feeling much better and quickly resumed her work at the election campaign office, for the voting was to take place on 21 February. Unfortunately, after just a few days, her back began to bother her again and despite her reluctance to relinquish her Labour Party work, she agreed that it was probably better to sit it out at home and convalesce there.

She consoled herself by having me display large election posters on behalf of the Labour candidate along the full length of our front garden and in so doing we upset most of the village. I had positioned each poster so that even speeding motorists could not fail to see them and the incredulous working-class villagers, overwhelmed by our boldness, mentioned in hushed tones that it was the first time they had ever seen a Labour poster displayed in Langley Burrell. The middle-class representatives, all Conservatives, let it be known that to flaunt a socialist poster outside an elegant house like ours was simply not done. This was to be expected in a hierarchical village such as Langley Burrell where workmen still touched their caps with respect whenever they were greeted by the squire, who still owned most of their homes and farmlands. Of course the posters did not make the slightest difference to the result of the election – it was an intractably safe Conservative seat – but we felt definitely chirpy in that we may have encouraged other faint-hearts to put up left-wing posters in the future. Jean positvely guffawed in bed when I related the backwash our front garden publicity was creating and she itched to be out campaigning on the streets.

However, she continued to be plagued by severe pain in her back which made any kind of sitting position virtually impossible. 'My back's locked,' she would plead and the discomfort did not let up at all. Doctors diagnosed it as a strain triggered off by the influenza and the strenuous walk to the bird sanctuary. As the pain became more regular however and the weeks dragged on I suspected that it might indicate something more insidious than mere strain. I did not pass on my apprehensions to Jean who continued to be confident and typically sanguine. 'I ricked my back going across the fields that day and it will get better if I rest,' she would explain to friends. 'I must learn to be patient and I'll be better in no time.'

During our months of attending Tuesday auctions, Jean and I

developed a craze for collecting old bits of farm machinery from the era when farm work was done by horses. When a farmer friend, Bill Fry, mentioned that he knew someone at the nearby village of Corsham who was leaving their farmhouse and wished to sell the contents, we were keen to have first crack at buying them. We arranged to see the goods on Sunday afternoon and Bill, Jean and I drove to Corsham together. I could see that Jean was still not well but she was weary of staying in bed and insisted on accompanying us to the farm. The pain in her back continued to persist, making it difficult for her to walk, and she made a hasty assessment of the contents. However, I was slightly heartened by seeing her run out of a hay barn after being confronted by a large rat. She and I agreed to purchase everything for a reasonable price and as soon as we had made the necessary transactions with the farmer I took Jean home since I could see that she was extremely tired.

I continued the drive from Langley Burrell to the next village to drop Bill off. On the way there I suggested that we stop at a pub so that I could repay him for his kindness with a drink. Bill was a rough diamond in his sixties who had made a lot of money as a cattle dealer and was not accustomed to pulling his punches; as soon as we sat down with our drinks he remarked, 'Jean's a nice woman. I really like her a lot.' I thanked him for the compliment but as he drained his beer he added, 'What's wrong with her?'

Without even reflecting on an answer I replied like an automaton, 'She's had cancer and I think it's coming back.' Frankly, I was quite astonished at my own words, for this was the first time I had openly acknowledged to anyone – including myself – that I suspected that the disease had returned. Probably it was easier to say it to Bill, a new and casual friend, than to someone close to me and, in a depressing haze of growing recognition, I appreciated the straightforwardness which prodded me into waking up to the full reality of the situation. (Two months later Bill was to drop dead while making an early morning cup of tea; we had lost a good neighbour.)

Within the next few weeks, Jean's back became even more bothersome and we began a series of regular weekly trips to the Churchill Hospital in Oxford. The doctors revealed nothing to Jean about her condition and, while her spirits were good, she

37

complained to me that the medical staff became evasive whenever she inquired about the nature of her illness. Their reticence caused her to suspect that something was seriously wrong and her anxiety I found hard to allay because I simply did not know the facts or theories which the doctors were considering. With the mastectomy not far behind us, I could hardly tell Jean that there was no possibility of cancer and I soon exhausted alternative explanations. Our relationship over twenty-one years had flourished on an understanding of frankness and honesty but I now felt considerable strain on my part, as if I were participating in a conspiracy designed to withhold the true diagnosis at any cost.

Although I was hard at work launching the book written at Wells (*Passports and Politics*) through press conferences and radio interviews as well as doing a special investigation for the *Sunday Times*, I became obsessed with Jean's health and decided to take steps to find out precisely what was wrong. Obviously no one was going to tell me. When Jean and I were preparing for another trip to Oxford, I asked her to tell the doctors that I insisted on seeing them for a short talk after they had finished their examinations. She was keen to cooperate as she felt that I might make the break-through where she had failed. The situation evoked memories of our previous experiences at Southend General Hospital when the first signs of cancer had appeared. Jean used to attend the consultant's clinic well in time for her appointments but would find herself being called after later arrivals, often being the last patient to be seen. She began to suspect that the doctor was embarrassed at having to impart grim news. Certainly a doctor's reluctance to be honest with a fatally ill patient is justifiable if he feels that frankness will do irreparable harm to the patient's peace of mind, but in Jean's case absolutely no effort was made to assess her ability to cope with the truth. I found it incredible that there were no skilled ancillary workers to assess the patient's emotional needs at such a crucial point. I found it even more astonishing that not one member of the medical staff, either at Southend and Oxford, expressed a desire to talk to me despite the fact that I was always visible and available to them during scores of hospital visits. In desperation I decided that I must confront them with my need to know the unqualified truth.

After returning to Oxford for her next check-up, Jean told her doctor that I wanted to speak with one of the medical staff about her case. Eventually I was summoned by a nurse into an office where I found a woman physician in her thirties behind her desk. From the outset of the conversation, her nervousness and reluctance to speak openly gave me no alternative but to ask unequivocally for the truth, emphasizing that I was responsible for family happiness and it was unfair that we should have to continue in such agonizing ignorance. 'How my wife faces up to the news is my affair,' I told the doctor, 'and you owe it to both of us to tell me what the situation is. What none of you seem to realize is that the mere lack of information is causing us more worry than necessary.'

After a long pause, the doctor weighed her words extremely carefully, 'It looks as if the cancer has come back. We don't know where it is or what part of the body is affected because the pain seems to be travelling. But I should warn you that the situation is very serious and you should prepare yourself to expect the worst.'

At these words, I had to swallow hard to prevent myself from breaking down on the spot. I managed to mumble that this was not a complete surprise because of the history of cancer in Jean's family and that Jean was afraid she was going to die of lung cancer as her mother had in 1967. I thanked the doctor for her help and stumbled into the corridor quite overwhelmed, but I had to pull myself together because I knew that within seconds I might be face-to-face with Jean. Haunted by these words, which sounded the death-knell for her as far as I could see, I could no longer fool myself as to what lay ahead for Jean and me, but what was I to tell her? Mercifully she was still under examination somewhere else in the hospital. I returned to the cubicle where we had parted and sat down, turning over in my mind a course of action. I reasoned with myself that I could limit the information to half-truths by relating to Jean only part of the content of the interview, hedging it with qualifications such as the doctors did not know anything for certain, that it might be a mild form of cancer or, than again, it might be something else. I rehearsed my speech for the ten minutes before Jean appeared and when she returned naturally her first words were, 'What did they say?'

I offered my amended version of the interview, improvising with a lot of my own ideas. I stressed that she was ill, that she should be fully aware that something was wrong, but that she should not necessarily accept the possibility that it was cancer. With mild pain-killers, she would still be able to get about. She appeared to accept this explanation with few qualms and after she had dressed I suggested that we have a nice lunch somewhere and do some shopping in Swindon before returning home. I had learned that action was a great palliative for Jean, as it was with me, and this was the strategy I was to adopt endless times in the next few months. We enjoyed a steak at a pub outside Farringdon, washing it down with a bottle of wine. Jean seemed happy, which helped restore my equilibrium. We discussed our plans for a holiday and our ideas for a private hotel while chuckling intermittently over two ponies at the pub window gazing hungrily at the diners. Neither of us made any reference to the illness. I had begun to appreciate that with a situation like the one we were facing, you simply cannot dwell on it or you invite madness. In order to survive you must become, if you are not already, an escapist.

That Easter we decided to spend a few days in Bournemouth, staying with my Aunt Stella, and so take the opportunity to see my brother Garth's new yacht which he was about to launch at the sailing club where my father was commodore. It was a crisp, sunny morning when Jean and I drove to the quay and she was eager to inspect the yacht while it was still on land. Half-way up the steep, six-rung ladder she could go no further. I could see how her back pained her but with lots of people around, mostly family, she put on a brave front. 'I just don't feel like getting in the boat,' she said gaily. 'My back's hurting a bit.' Virtually everyone present suspected the cancer was spreading yet no one made a fuss because they all knew how Jean hated having attention drawn to herself. We spent the rest of the day in the sailing club watching a giant crane lift dozens of yachts into the Blue Lagoon in Poole Harbour and their owners preparing them for a season's sailing.

The following day was plagued with rain but Jean fretted to go out so we went for a drive to the mouth of Poole Harbour to watch the ferry boat and the tramp steamers. While we sat in the car at the water's edge I could see that Jean was in acute discomfort but she refused my pleas to take her back to bed and said she would rather remain there. Following my conversation with the doctor a week earlier, the consequences of the illness began to assault me with quite an impact. I could no longer close my eyes to just how sick Jean was. Being confined in the car with her that day, watching such acute agony at close quarters, made me realize that we had reached a frightening impasse. As we sat in silence, the horror of it all began to hit me in such a way that parts of me started to go out of control. I made an excuse to get out of the car by offering to buy some chocolates and I was grateful when Jean agreed that she was a bit hungry. After a brief visit to the confectionary shop, I became so choked that, in desperation, I ran into an empty phone booth where I wept and wept, the first time I had cried since my initial meeting with the doctor in Oxford. I could no longer deny to myself that Jean was dying. Moments passed. I continued to cry until I realized that Jean would be wondering where I was. I made an effort to pull myself together, running back to the car with my face turned upwards in order to drench myself in rain and I stuffed a chocolate bar in my mouth to camouflage the stifled feeling in my throat. Jean did not appear to notice anything strange about me and when I suggested that we go to a movie that evening she said she was quite enthusiastic. Just before leaving the phone kiosk I had noticed an advertisement for 'The Sting' which both Jean and I had wanted to see so she took a few more pain-killers and we drove into Bournemouth to divert ourselves with a pleasant evening at the movies. We returned to Chippenham the following day, resuming our leisurely routine, rarely alluding to the disconcerting pains which continued to plague Jean with alarming intensity and frequency.

5 PORTENTS

One of the quirks of being a newspaper reporter is that many of the things one has to write about can touch closely on one's own life. Not long after Jean and I returned from Bournemouth, the news desk asked me to go to Coventry to write an article on the memorial service for Richard Crossman, the former Labour Cabinet Minister. I had met him briefly a few months earlier at an election meeting in Birmingham and I noted how ill he looked. A colleague had told me at the time that Crossman was dying of cancer. Two months later, here I was reporting on his death rites in a most uncomfortable assignment but one which I could not refuse.

As Mrs Crossman entered Coventry Cathedral which was resounding with awesome organ music, I could not help identifying with her. I felt myself becoming shaky. I wanted to flee. In order to escape the most depressing thoughts, I made copious notes on the service and the cathedral, almost all of which were unnecessary. Would I be like this in a few months' time, grieving like Mrs Crossman? When the service ended I wandered out into Coventry and over a cup of tea in a café I wrote a disjointed account of the proceedings which I telephoned to the office before I started the long drive home.

In the car, driving through the bleak fog and intermittent rain, I reflected on how unsettling it was to be reminded of the inevitable conclusion to Jean's struggle with cancer. I realized how important it was not to dwell on the reality of death. To do so would encourage a sense of utter futility and undermine whatever spiritual resolve remained. When I arrived in Chippenham, depressed and discouraged, I was mightily relieved to find Jean perky and well, having just arranged a dinner party for the following evening with Aunt Gwen in Bristol. Seeing this, I began to believe in life again and Jean, as if intuiting this, reported to the guests at the dinner party in a loud and clear voice that apart from a few back pains, she was really quite well. It was a most enjoyable evening and I pushed the Crossman incident as much into obscurity as my mind would allow.

A few weeks later we went to a farm auction in Sutton Benger where Jean spotted a pretty oak dressing table which we decided to bid for. Unfortunately, it was listed as one of the last items in the auction and we would have some time to wait. Jean began to feel the strain of standing for such a long period and went to sit in the car for the hour's wait. I managed to buy the piece for five pounds so I loaded it into the boot of the car and we drove home, satisfied with our little acquisition. Jean mentioned how she looked forward to acquiring many more things but, with the spells of pain increasing in frequency, this was in fact the last auction she attended.

However, it was important for us to continue believing in the future and we pursued our plans with an iron will. After a fallow period in which I had done no book writing – mainly because of house moving and hospital visiting – I managed to sell my idea for a biography of Michael de Freitas, alias Michael X, the Black Power leader in Britain during the 1960s to Hart-Davis, MacGibbon, the London publishers. Jean was keen to help with the research in any possbile way. She had agreed to shelve plans for the hotel and we intended to start work on the book as soon as I had more free time at home. It happened at this particular time that the political situation in Northern Ireland worsened considerably – it was the spring of 1974 – and as one of the team of *Sunday Times* reporters assigned to cover events there, I had to pay frequent visits to write about shootings, bombings, and general political instability. I was usually away from dawn on Wednesday until Sunday, when Edgar or Clive would drive to Heathrow

Airport to collect me after an early morning flight from Belfast. Jean's equanimity was tested after the first week of the Ulster Workers' Council strike in May of that year when I was involved in an incident which was potentially dangerous. While driving through the Bogside, the IRA stronghold in Londonderry, I was stopped by three armed men at a checkpoint. They said they needed my rented car because it had an English registration number and they demanded my driving licence as well. I was thus 'kidnapped' and left with a guard until later in the evening when the car was finally returned to me intact. I was not unduly unnerved by the incident but annoyed that an entire day had been wasted and I was anxious to telephone Jean to see how she was. When my call reached Chippenham she seemed well and happy so I deliberately withheld news of my kidnapping, hoping to put the experience in the past. However, when I returned to London, the news desk asked me to write a short account of my misadventure and I reluctantly did so, knowing that there was no concealing my fate from Jean now. On the following Sunday as we sat in the garden at Pinchloafe reading the papers I saw out of the corner of my eye that Jean had noticed the story with the headling 'Reporter Hijacked by IRA'. I expected a reaction of chagrin or incredulity and was immensely relieved when she commented in the most casual way, 'Oh, is that what happens to you in Ireland then!' She showed remarkable composure yet again when the news desk phoned within an hour instructing me to return to Londonderry immediately because airline pilots were threatening to shut down flights to Belfast. So, after three hours at home, I was off again to troubled Ireland.

Ulster was in such a state of paralysis that it was difficult for a visitor to survive. I returned to the same hotel outside Londonderry which I had used the previous week only to find it on the verge of closing. After some persuasion, they agreed that I could have a room but there would be no service of any sort because the staff was either on strike or afraid to work. In the evenings I managed to get across the border for a meal as well as to telephone home. I was disconcerted by bad news from Vivienne when I telephoned Chippenham on Thursday evening: apparently Jean was in

45

considerable pain and confined to bed. However, Vivienne assured me that the doctor was in attendance and everything was under control. I promised to return in two days' time instead of the three I had planned and I hastened to complete my article the following day, phoning it to the office in the late afternoon.

I found myself with an evening to kill so I invited another journalist, David White of the *Financial Times*, who had joined me at the hotel, to visit two old friends, Ray and Sheila McLean. Ray, a doctor in the Bogside, was just ending his term of office as Mayor of Londonderry, the first Catholic to hold that office despite the predominantly Catholic population of the town. The opportunity to have good food and drink with stimulating company would, I hoped, divert me from my growing preoccupation with Jean's worsening condition. However, as the conversation at the McLean's flowed, I became progressively withdrawn. It was beginning to dawn on me how frequently Jean's crises were occurring and I kept asking myself how rapidly the deterioration was going to progress, and when and how it would end.

Very gently, Ray prodded my thoughts and I told him how worried I was about Jean, whom he had never met. I provided him with a brief synopsis of her illness to put him in the picture and I could not resist asking him, 'How serious do you think it is?' It may have seemed a naïve question but I realize now that at that stage I had still not fully accepted the diagnosis that the cancer had returned. Ray's answer was hushed but devastatingly straight-forward. He warned me, 'She's not going to recover because no one does from that kind of situation.' He added ominously, 'You've got to accept that she's going to die, Derek.'

It was not the surprise so much as the overt confirmation of the dreaded suspicion that bowled me over. I left the room, sat on the staircase and broke down. Ray, who waited a while for my feelings to subside, came to the stairs and tried to console me by presenting me with a wooden Madonna which he wanted me to pass on to Jean. I told him what he already knew, that neither Jean nor I was religious but he insisted, saying, 'Take it to her anyway, it will probably help her.'

The gift was a curious incident. Here was Ray, a leader of the Catholic people in a city devastated by civil war, a doctor who sees death frequently, giving an atheist a cherished symbol of his

46

religion. Although Ray and I had known one another for years, I realized then that in spiritual matters we were poles apart. At that point I was sorely disillusioned with life and had almost ceased to believe in anything. In my grief I could not fully acknowledge the gesture of fellowship which Ray so obviously intended. I found the gift embarrassing and I could only harbour cynical feelings about graven images; I pocketed it so as not to appear impolite but I had every intention of forgetting about it. I never had the heart to give it to Jean because I feared that, even with her distrust of religion, she might see the gift of the Madonna as an ill omen. I realize now that this was a well-meaning gesture and I regret that I did not properly acknowledge it. Perhaps subconsciously I resented his plain speaking and refused to forgive him for robbing me of my few illusions.

After the incident with the Madonna I recovered sufficiently to re-join the little party and I was immensely relieved when we proceeded to drink for the entire night, solving most of Ireland's political problems, emerging at 6 A.M. very much the worse for wear. We behaved giddily and irresponsibly: I climbed on the bonnet of my car pretending to have passed out, which led to further horse-play between us. Finally David dragged me off and we drove very shakily through deserted streets back to our hotel on the other side of the city.

I packed my bag in a frenzied hurry and set out again on the eighty-mile drive to Belfast Airport in order to catch the London plane. As I crossed the mountains on a cold, bright morning, I debated whether to go straight home from the airport or to keep a speaking appointment at a conference on racial harmony in London. I delayed the decision until my hangover had subsided and we had reached London; when we touched down at Heathrow, I rang home right away for a report on Jean's condition. It seemed that she was neither better nor worse and that a few hours either way would make little difference. I decided to honour my commitment to the conference and I relayed the message to Jean that I would be home by tea-time.

I made a short speech to the conference, apologizing for the inadequacy of my talk by saying that I had been reporting in Ulster for two solid weeks. The audience easily appreciated this since the province was the focus of national attention at that time.

47

I could not tell them the truth that it was all I could manage to carry out my *Sunday Times* work as well as worry about and care for Jean. Normally, even under pressure, I would have written that speech either on the air flight or in the corner of a bar without any undue bother, and these increasing lapses in my ability to carry out my professional obligations caused my self-respect to take a disturbing plunge.

When I returned to Chippenham I discovered that the local doctor had arranged for Jean to be taken back to Oxford on Monday. The pain had 'localized' itself to the extent that it was hoped that the experts could finally identify its real source. I was equally anxious that the uncertainty be removed so that treatment could be more specific. Before leaving the farmhouse, Jean had to be heavily drugged so that she could endure the agony of being lifted from bed to stretcher and into the ambulance for the long journey ahead. I accompanied her on the ride and noted that, mercifully, she slept most of the way.

We stopped at Malmesbury to pick up a woman of about fifty who was due for a routine check-up at the hospital. She was anxious to talk to someone and as we cruised through the countryside she related to me how she had had a breast removed several months earlier and this was one of her regular visits for radiotherapy. I was struck by her gay manner, her self-confidence, and her final remark that, 'Only two more visits and I'll be fit to go back to work.' Jean continued to sleep during our conversation and the woman nodded her head in Jean's direction as she finally asked the question I had been dreading, 'What's wrong with your wife?' The similarity between this woman's condition and Jean's twelve months previously made me pause in confusion. I had no right to destroy this woman's ebullience by describing Jean's medical history which was all too like her own.

'She's not very well,' I replied cryptically, steadfastly refusing to say more. I noticed the poor woman looking accusingly at me for not exchanging confidences as she had done but I knew that, however bad-mannered I appeared, I was right to keep quiet. Perhaps under less stressful conditions I might have been able to talk to her more tactfully without disturbing her peace of mind. Unfortunately, the sight of her brimming gaiety and determination was a grim reminder of Jean's former self and I found myself enormously saddened by the encounter.

When we arrived in Oxford, Jean's consultant decided to keep her at the hospital for a few days in order to administer a battery of tests. Jean had half expected this and had brought her overnight case with her. I found her genuinely pleased over the ensuing series of tests; she remarked as we said good-bye, 'We'll soon know what it is and then we can do something about it.' In fact she remained in the hospital for a week and the results were to be known perhaps a week or ten days after that.

I could see that, despite overwhelming odds, Jean and I were still clinging to the hope that her illness was not cancer. Even after my conversations with the doctor in Oxford and Ray McLean in Londonderry, I continued to hope that their diagnoses would prove to be wrong. Jean and I confined our attention to the few cases of cancer where the disease, even if it had not been cured, had regressed. 'There are plenty of instances where cancer has just stopped, although for what reason we don't really know,' was a favourite comment made by doctors at the time. This possibility, however tenuously backed by statistical evidence, provided us with the one straw of hope we so desperately needed.

Jean and I had always been blessed with good fortune in our life together and obviously I was banking on an extension of our good luck. On the surface, my philosophy was to tell as few people as possible about the real situation, carry on as normally as I could, keep Jean buoyant on a day-to-day basis, and never let my guard slip for a moment. In Jean's presence this was not such a difficult task; her self-possession and sanguinity were so infectious it was always a pleasure to visit her in the hospital, despite her being in a ward in which some thirty people were suffering from cancer. However, every few days someone would die and I would leave the ward with a premonition of the fate awaiting Jean. Especially during the long and sleepless nights I would turn over and over in my mind all the horrific possibilities of the disease and wonder what on earth was going to happen to us.

Just before returning to Chippenham, Jean realized that she would be confined to bed for some time and she felt she would rather move downstairs in the farmhouse. Knowing that it would be good for her to be in close touch with the rest of the family, I made up a bed in the breakfast room so that she could see past her favourite rose bushes to the end of the rear garden. By now it was late May and there was an abundance of colour. I prepared another bed for myself alongside Jean's and when she arrived home, she was delighted with our living quarters. She quickly settled into her new life with plenty of people to talk to; family were frequently passing through and there was a telephone within close reach. The kitchen was adjacent to the breakfast room so that she could easily shout instructions about food preparation and cooking schedules.

Our G.P. called every Monday as a matter of routine. During his first call after Jean's return, Dr Gornall asked the usual questions and conducted the customary examination before repeating prescriptions for all her drugs. Both Jean and I knew that the second call was far more important since by then the results of the Oxford tests would have been confirmed and sent on to Chippenham. When Dr Gornall did appear for his second visit, he said nothing at all to Jean apart from the routine questioning about her daily health but as I showed him out he muttered to me, 'Can I talk to you for a moment?'

It was the dreaded moment. The truth would be mine, whether I liked it or not. We walked down the drive towards his car and I sensed that he was gathering his wits in order to say something crucial. When he spoke, his words were not entirely unexpected although nonetheless they provided me with quite a blow. 'I've had the results from Oxford,' he said quietly. 'The cancer has spread to the bone and you must expect your wife to be dead by the end of the year.'

Seven months of life left. That was all she had. I leaned against his car and gazed through the front gate at nothing in particular. I had little, if anything, to say. When Dr Gornall went on to suggest the means of treatment in the last stages of Jean's illness, I felt a sudden flush of anger.

'When the end comes near, we can take your wife into the local cottage hospital where she will be well looked after,' he pointed out.

'Absolutely not,' I retorted. 'She'd rather die at home. It doesn't matter how much trouble it is, we'll look after her ourselves providing you'll come and keep the pain under control.'

'Of course I will,' he answered sympathetically, obviously understanding how important it was that we should share the final days together.

I asked him to explain what bone cancer was and he replied that the cancer had started in her left breast and then spread in a secondary way into the bone. The disease gradually eats away the marrow, edging its way towards the bone's surface; as it emerges near this surface the area becomes extremely painful. (Jean later came to label these areas as her 'pain-spots'.) At this point, the outbreaks were concentrated in the pelvic and thigh regions.

After stressing that I was to call on him at any time to alleviate whatever discomforts should arise, Dr Gornall drove off and I sat on the low wall in the drive to think things over. What was I to tell Jean? Once in the past when she had suspected that I was having a clandestine talk with the doctor, she had been quick to tax me about it despite the fact that her suspicions were unfounded. However, she well knew that on this particular visit the doctor had brought with him the results of the laboratory tests from Oxford. Having heard his car drive off a full fifteen minutes after he had said good-bye to her would confirm in her mind that he and I had been talking.

I walked back to the house using the long route around the garages and passed her window, waving with a forced cheerfulness at her and I emerged in the kitchen via the conservatory. When I finally reached her bedside she confronted me with the inevitable question: 'What did the doctor tell you?' I still had no clear idea what to say so I fenced the issue by saying, 'We only discussed how to look after you. There are still lots of tests to be done and we've got to keep on nursing you and looking after you.' I said this as casually as possible but I could see that my improvised explanation was not impressing her much. Stalling for more time, I suggested that we have some tea and I went into the kitchen. When I returned to the sickroom she asked again, 'What *did* the doctor say? Derek, I think you're holding back on me and I want to know the truth. Whatever the news is, I'd rather you told me.'

I realized then that I could no longer withhold anything from her. However, for the first time in our relationship, I hadn't the heart to look her straight in the face so, staring at the side of the bed, I said, 'The doctors say that you have bone cancer.'

51

'How long will I have to live?' she asked instantly.

Still staring at the bedpost, I said almost inaudibly, 'They say until about the end of the year.'

'Oh,' was all she said for the rest of the day.

Jean remained silent and unmoving not only that afternoon and evening but for the whole of the following day as well. I brought her food to eat and water to wash with, rituals she endured as if by rote. She did not read any of the morning or evening papers which I placed on her bedside table nor did she listen to the radio at all. I could tell she did not want to speak so I merely sat, intent and immovable, watching her withdraw into an impenetrable shell, staring through the window at the long back garden. Whenever I put my arms around her and made any attempt to console her, I was met with silence. By now I was quite terrified, fearing that I had done the wrong thing in telling her the truth and I was full of self-reproach. Was she going to will herself to death? Was the torment of being sentenced to death too great for her?

In spite of my remorse, I tried to keep things going fairly normally, making the meals, dealing with callers, doing a quick stint in the garden, but never leaving her out of my sight for more than a few minutes. I found it intolerable sitting in the same room all the time with my conscience hammering away at me, condemning me for having robbed Jean of whatever peace of mind remained to her.

The third day began again in silence. I got up early, telephoned the office to say that I would not come to work, and made the breakfast. When I carried the tray into the sick-room, I decided to continue with a surface appearance of normality and I greeted Jean with, 'Good morning, love, how are you?' expecting pained silence as my only reply. However, she turned towards me and spoke, choosing her words very carefully. 'I'm all right now,' she said slowly. 'I've thought about everything and I'll be all right. It's quite obvious that I'll have to accept all this so I'm just going to make the best of it.'

My relief at this point was so great that I lapsed into speechlessness, overjoyed in the knowledge that I had not misjudged Jean after all. What she had needed was time to think things out and emerge from the first awful sense of shock; I could see that in effect she had been in mourning for herself. Her mood was sombre but she did radiate an air of inner calm as she spoke of the state of domestic disrepair which she could only blame on the excess of attention lavished on her in the preceding weeks. She dictated a shopping list, reminding me of the many odd calls to be made, and with painstaking care recommended which shops in Chippenham I should go to. More relieved than anything else, I joyously obeyed all her requests and when Edgar came in I asked him to sit with Jean while I went out on my various errands.

I drove away from the farmhouse towards Chippenham reflecting on the courage of this woman who was making her peace with death. And, of course, there was self-interest on my part as well. Jean's courage and fortitude made it so much easier for me to care for her. I was aware that she had clearly thought of this.

The next few days were a period of profound depression for us both. Not a depression of petulance or anger but an awareness of the separation to come. How would it end? I told the family that Jean had bone cancer from which she would not recover; for that matter, I told anyone else who was interested. We did not parade our tragedy but at the same time there was no point in being secretive about it. People received the news with a kind of calm shock – most of them had seen it coming. Many friends and colleagues wrote me private letters expressing their concern. Harold Evans, the editor of the *Sunday Times*, wrote to express his regret and say that I need not return to work until the problem was resolved.

Since breaking her silence Jean made every effort to exude good spirits, making sure that anyone who called at Pinchloafe also came to see her, behaving as if there were nothing untoward about the household. Inwardly we were both suffering a good deal: Jean over being sentenced to death in the prime of life and myself over the fact that I was going to lose her. However, she refused to surrender to grief or tears. Instead she concentrated her energies on planning a new life for me. It was in the first week of the bombshell news that she first suggested that I marry again after her death. 'Promise me you will marry again,' she would say. 'I'd like that. There are plenty of women in the world looking for a husband.' She even mentioned the names of a few unattached women we knew but I had no stomach for this kind of speculation and shrank into an appalled state of embarrassment. 'Yes, I expect I'll marry again,' I would tell her. 'But I don't really want to talk about it. My only concern for the time being is you.'

'I wish you'd not had that vasectomy,' she grieved. She could not bring herself to make the other half of the statement, which was that I might want to have children by another woman.

I reassured her that I was not over-anxious to have another family and, anyway, I could have a repair job. 'They're making big advances in perfecting repair surgery for vasectomies,' I told her, 'and I think doctors emphasize the difficulty in repair to discourage people from lightly going into vasectomy. I feel sure that in a case like mine the medical profession would do its utmost.' That seemed to console her.

If it was helping to relieve her burden then I was happy to go along with her but my heart was never in it. It would always be a rather one-sided conversation, ending with her commenting, 'You'll get over losing me – and you'll find another wife and be happy again.' It was not that I disagreed with her, for I silently realized that I would have to survive the loss and find another mate eventually. However, talking about this face-to-face with my still attractive wife was unendurable for me. It was so like Jean, in any tough situation, to make contingency plans so that others would suffer less. Perhaps thinking that she was herself preparing me for a life without her and herself prodding me into it relieved her own stress. I chose to believe that.

It has been said that we have the strength to bear the misfortunes of others and by a strange coincidence the problems of a number of people close to us alleviated our own burden considerably. Someone else has said that he who finds himself resolves his own misery and I am convinced that Jean in her role of counsellor, therapist, and listener, was at her strongest at this particular time. The first blow came with the breakdown of Edgar and Vivienne's marriage, just six months after they had wed. It had been stormy for some time, which was not surprising considering their extreme youthfulness, and a crisis occurred just two days after Jean had broken her silence. After a heated argument, Vivienne had left Edgar in a huff and disappeared for several days. When Vivienne reappeared – reluctantly – Jean spent many hours talking to both of them on their own, trying to help them understand the reasons for the marital breakdown. After long discussions over several days, it was eventually agreed by the two youngsters to accept an offer from Vivienne's father to spend a long working holiday on his charter yacht in the south of France. When they flew off to the sun a week later, their mood was far more constructive and Jean and I were hopeful. I was happy to see Jean so involved in the reconciliation since it gave her a sense of mission in life. Gradually the phone calls from the Riviera took on a more optimistic note and we were much relieved that the rift was healing.

After they were gone there were new distractions, since I was forced to take full responsibility for Edgar's extremely time-consuming business of selling reconditioned gear-boxes and transmission systems. As it happened, he had just conducted a massive mail-order drive and Jean and I were reduced to handling dozens of phone calls each day from engineers, mechanics, automobile enthusiasts and the like, asking endless questions about gear-boxes. We developed a routine of diplomatically stalling those callers whose questions foxed us and invited others to come and visit the 'showroom' (in fact, one of Edgar's garages) if the catalogue showed that the gear-box they needed was in stock. We became quite urbane in our sales talk although there were inevitable *faux pas* committed in the presence of some all-knowing car mechanics. Once potential customers were on our doorstep I would lead them into the showroom, point them in the direction of the rows of transmission systems and say, 'Well, it's here, but you'll have to find it.' Fortunately, we were lucky in selling to professionals who needed little guidance and I was quite proud that under our management the business remained intact and even made a small profit.

Another problem emerged with Vivienne's thirteen-year-old brother, Jeremy, who had been living with us with a view to becoming part of the family. He enjoyed staying with us and we were very fond of him but I was fearful that Jean might deteriorate quickly at any moment, needing all my attention. I did not want to neglect Jeremy for long periods at a time although he was a resourceful and self-sufficient boy. Jean and I agreed that to delay in telling him would only make things harder for him so one afternoon in the garden I explained that Jean was dying and because of this he would have to leave and go back to live with his grandmother. His disappointment and distress were apparent but he sympathized with our dilemma and agreed that there was no alternative but to leave. He enjoyed his grandmother's home but he obviously preferred our younger family. 'Can I come back and spend some weekends with you?' he asked, and I said how delighted both Jean and I would be to see him again.

Just after I had spoken with Jeremy, we heard news of Irvine, the West Indian boy whom we had last seen at Christmas. Apparently he had suffered a mild nervous breakdown caused by isolation and excessive studying; he had been preparing for his 'O' level examinations in the hopes that, upon completion, he would take up a post as junior reporter which I had arranged for him but which post was conditional on his securing four 'O' levels. Unfortunately, Irvine had tried too hard, working from a lonely bed-sitting room in a more desolate part of London without enough human contact and relaxation, and a few days before the examinations he had suffered a temporary breakdown. Had I not been so preoccupied with Jean, I would normally have spent more time with him and perhaps seen the collapse coming. Now the most I could do was to find someone to take care of Jean for the day while I drove to London to visit Irvine in the hospital. I was able to report back to Jean that I had seen him and his psychiatrist and that there was no doubt of his recovery after sufficient rest.

As if this was not enough, my brother's marriage began to fall apart. Both Garth and his wife came to see Jean and I on several occasions that month to discuss their troubles but the rift was too great to be repaired and eventually they separated. Jean and I were struck by the fact that we lived in a world of other people's troubles, with the difference that, on the whole, theirs were resolvable whereas ours were not. However, Jean in particular realized that immersing herself in these preoccupations helped her to temporarily forget her own fate. By concentrating our energies on counselling others, we did not have the opportunity to brood excessively over our own lives. Thus, ironically, as the pressures from others initially distracted us and gradually began to ease away, Jean and I went through a period of extraordinary calm and togetherness. It was a lovely summer and occasionally Jean would get out in the garden for a few minutes and walk among the flowers. We were making the most of what time we had left together; the depression had eased into a stoic acceptance of the fate we could not avoid. We were merely coasting along, savouring the present moments, refusing to capitulate to tears or anguish as much for one another's sake as for our own.

However, I did have to practise great caution about what I said. Too blatant reminders of the future – the cancer and its inevitable course – could not be entirely accepted by Jean. That summer I accepted all the cooking duties, guided by her instructions which she would holler to me in the kitchen from the adjacent sick-room. One evening I was doing particularly well at the stove and carelessly I called back to Jean, 'I'll soon be a good cook at this rate.' When I finished my task, I strolled into her room to find her in tears. When I asked her what the matter was she replied, 'It's because you're learning to live without me.' I could have bitten my tongue off. It was a warning signal that I must be extremely cautious about any comments, never dwelling on anything that indicated what the future would be like for me without Jean.

Yet I could not entirely escape from speculations about how I was going to cope on my own. Other people seemed curiously concerned with my contingency plans and it surprised me how frequently I was asked, 'What are you going to do when Jean is dead?' or 'Are you going to sell the farmhouse afterwards?' I resented these questions. They were premature and certainly in bad taste and I considered that the answers were my business, not theirs. Thus I developed a stock reply which I refused to elaborate on: 'I shall leave everything as it is for a year after her death and then decide what to do.' This strategy was to reassure the children as much as anything, for they had thrown their lot in with us in moving to Wiltshire and naturally they wondered about their future.

Jean and I continued to concentrate on the present and I was impressed by how effectively she had pushed the fatal prognosis into some rarely visited recess of her mind. This was typified by her behaviour during a visit from two of her girlfriends who came down on the train from London to spend the day with her. I kept

57

clear most of the time in order that the three of them could have a good chin-wag; they chatted happily all day and after tea I drove the two women to the railway station to put them on the evening train back to London. During the ride one of them said out of the blue, 'I just can't understand it. Does she know how ill she is?'

'She knows she is going to die,' I replied.

During the whole of the visit , Jean had not mentioned her health or the fact that she was not expected to live more than six months. Her two friends were both baffled and marvelling. When I arrived home Jean remarked on what a splendid day they had spent together and how much she hoped they would come again. Avoiding any mention of the real reason why they had come was her own special way of transcending the situation.

6 THE PACT

For many weeks things were so calm at home that we began to wonder if the doctors were wrong. When I had first been given the news about the certainty of the bone cancer, I had the feeling that life was going to be pure hell from that moment on but there we were, actually enjoying the summer. The doctors at Oxford had exuded confidence saying, 'There's a long way to go yet,' and Jean was investing all her energies and enthusiasm in this possibility. She began to plan for a long convalescence, sending me out to buy all those magazines which specialised in advertising living-in home helps. She planned to offer someone the cottage rent-free in exchange for helping to look after her, and she needed the magazines to evaluate the market in a field about which we knew nothing.

'I want you to go back to work,' she declared, for in fact I had done no writing for the *Sunday Times* in more than two months. 'All I need is someone to look after me and the self-contained cottage is a plum attraction.' Thus, during the afternoons while Jean slept, I spent my time restoring the cottage as close to its seventeenth-century appearance as I possibly could, removing all room partitions and fireplaces put in during Victorian times. With my efforts it began to assume a more elegant air, helped considerably by a natural stone fireplace I had built by a local craftsman.

While I was putting the finishing touches to the cottage Jean's father decided to return to Manchester to rejoin his friends and Vivienne and Edgar returned from the French Riviera looking brown and happy and obviously reconciled. They had made plans to rent a flat in a nearby village for a while as the cottage was still uninhabitable although Edgar continued to run his business from Pinchloafe House. It became such a halcyon period that Edgar and I, both needing more exercise, bought a two-seater touring canoe and we would paddle regularly in the evenings on the nearby river Avon while Vivienne sat with Jean. I managed to do some work for my newspaper by finding story ideas in the West Country and slipping away from home a few hours a day to gather information. Jean said how happy she would be to settle for a life like this which could go on indefinitely. Despite her diminished activities, it was a happy and cohesive time for us all. Our sense of well-being was further enhanced by the fact that we had finally sold our house in Billericay. This took a tremendous load off my mind.

However, our peace was abruptly shattered when, in the middle of August, areas of pain flared up in Jean's arm, leg, and back. There was no doubt that immediate hospitalization was necessary and when the ambulance arrived Jean knew she was in for a nightmare ride and swallowed as many pain-killers as she dared. However, the drugs could not entirely alleviate the discomfort and by the time we reached the hospital, she was crying out in distress. The only alleviations for Jean's condition was radio-therapy on the actual pain-spots but it was necessary to pinpoint these accurately by X ray beforehand. Additional pain-killers would have caused her to lose consciousness, thus preventing the radiographers from properly positioning her for their series of pictures. However, Jean became so convulsed with pain that she ceased having any control over her own movements; in just a few moments, she became so weak and distraught that I had to prop her up in front of the machine in different positions. The second the radiographers had finished, a doctor who had stood through-out poised with a syringe mercifully injected her with Pethedine and she passed out instantly.

During the next few days Jean deteriorated rapidly and had to be kept unconscious to relieve the pain. The consultant in charge explained that it was the pain rather than the cancer which was weakening her and at this rate she was not expected to live another week. Having seen the extent of her suffering on the day she came into the hospital, I was almost relieved to hear the verdict. I could not bear to think of her enduring that degree of pain again. At that point I began to accept that she was going to die and I began therefore to make some plans to deal with the event. My intention was to have her cremated quietly, issue a printed card informing everybody of what had happened, and flee for a while. I wanted to bolt in my car and keep running indefinitely, probably across Europe. I felt no inclination to share my grief with anyone else. Sitting at the bedside during all her unconscious hours gave me time to peruse several books of poetry for a suitable inscription to go on the card and I settled for the words by John Donne which best reflected my sentiments:

> All other things, to their destruction draw,
> Only our love hath no decay;
> This, no tomorrow hath, nor yesterday,
> Running it never runs from us away,
> But truly keeps his first, last, everlasting day.

However, despite my attempts to brace myself for Jean's death, my agony was in no way diminished at seeing the person I loved and adored wasting away in front of my eyes. Within a few days I was numb with the emotional stress and sleeplessness and I had to rely on my sons to drive me to Oxford to spend the afternoons and evenings at her bedside. Even my mornings were not free from stress for the telephone would ring constantly with relatives and friends inquiring about Jean. Eventually the unpleasantness of continually relating her condition to callers became too much for me and Vivienne took responsibility for all the calls. I simply waited for the end to come.

However, on the fifth day a miracle occurred. The medical staff – always careful, painstaking, sympathetic – had administered a new combination of drugs, a 'cocktail', which not only relieved Jean's pain but also allowed her to recover consciousness for an hour in the afternoon. During this entire time, I had witnessed the staff's intense involvement in Jean's suffering and my admiration for them knew no limit. I gathered from a doctor that during one fleeting instant of consciousness Jean had told the nurses that if she could not be conscious, she did not want to live, and I sensed that this remark of hers challenged them that much more in their determination to cope with this particular relapse. Whatever the truth, they succeeded after a number of different 'cocktails' had been administered and by that weekend Jean and I were able to talk to one another for short periods of time. At this point the doctors had switched the treatment from one of radiation menopause (essentially a taking away of hormones) to one of adding male hormones to Jean's system. This, together with the success in killing the pain, brought about a temporary recovery.

On the second day of Jean's return to consciousness, I came into the ward and noticed that she was propped up slightly and looking stronger. 'I'm not so dopey now,' she laughed as we kissed hello. I could see that she was making a big effort to fight off the residual effects of the massive doses of drugs which caused drowsiness and forgetfulness, and it became clear to me that she wanted to say something important. I pulled my chair closer to her and asked, 'Is there anything troubling you, dearest?'

'Derek,' she said, taking a deep breath, 'I simply don't want to go on living like this. It's been pretty bad this week and I want you to do something for me.'

As she paused a moment to gather her concentration, I promised I would do anything to help, as yet uncertain what it was. I asked her to go on.

'I want you to do something for me so that if I decide I want to die I can do it on my own terms and exactly when I choose. The one thing that worries me is that I won't be in any position to make the right decision, what with my being knocked senseless by all these drugs. I might be too daft to know whether I'm doing the right thing or not but I shall have a good idea when I've had enough of the pain. So I want you to promise me that when I ask you if this is the right time to kill myself, you will give me an honest answer one way or another and we must understand, both you and I, that I'll do it right at that very moment. You won't question my right and you will give me the means to do it.'

I was sobered but not entirely surprised at this request. Over the years Jean had often referred to the way in which her mother had died of lung cancer; she felt that her mother had suffered far too long because no one was willing to make a decision which would mercifully hasten the inevitable end. Jean would never refer to the incident in detail, too reticent to recount what had obviously been a traumatic experience for her, but I knew from the frequency with which she had alluded to her mother's horrible death that it was one of her worst recollections. She had resolved with a vengeance that such a fate would never befall her.

'If our positions were reversed,' I said to her, 'I know I would make the same request,' knowing this to be absolutely true. I had to reply finally, 'I'll do whatever you ask.'

Jean, as if to make sure she had made her point asked again, 'Do you promise that, when I ask the question, "Is this the end?" that you *will* give me the answer and then the means to carry it out?'

'Yes,' I replied, 'I promise, my darling,' holding on to both of her hands.

Apart from not wanting her to suffer unnecessarily, for I was almost as ravaged as she from the preceeding weeks' agony, I had to admire her decision and the strength of mind needed to make it. I rebelled at the thought of Jean's ever dying and a part of me strongly resisted being an accomplice; however, when the request for help in dying meant relief from relentless suffering and pain and I had seen the extent of this agony, the option simply could not be denied. I think that, finally, both my heart and mind had begun to accept the inevitability of Jean's dying. And certainly Jean deserved the dignity of selecting her own ending. She must die soon – as we both now realized – but together we would decide when this would be.

With my promise, Jean closed the subject and said she wanted to see Edgar who was waiting outside the ward. She and I never discussed the matter again. It was a covenant between man and wife – absolutely sacred to us – which she knew I had sealed with my promise. Driving home that night from the hospital, I told Edgar about his mother's request as much to test his reaction as to suggest that it was also a matter for the immediate family to be aware of and not solely my responsibility. Despite his maturity, he was overwhelmed by the complexity of it all although ultimately he gave a quiet assent. He respected his mother's sensibilities while realizing – as did I – that once Jean had made a decision, there was no dissuading her.

From that weekend on, Jean began to recover and within three weeks I was discussing with the doctors the possibility of bringing her home. Living in a cancer ward in which there is a steady succession of deaths was unbearably grim. One night I noticed that the bed opposite Jean was suddenly empty; when I asked her what had happened she told me that a young girl who was only twenty had died earlier in the day and I noticed how urgently Jean pressed me to get her out. 'I'm ready to come home now,' she implored.

When I spoke with the senior consultant, he agreed that home would be the best place for Jean because, as he put it, the will to live was the single most important factor in coping with the disease. He could plainly see that Jean wanted to be with her family. I asked him how long he thought she had to live and he replied, 'She still has a long way to go. She's tough and determined and there are still a number of drug treatments we can try.' I was encouraged by his words and when I told Jean she could come home in a few days, she was positively rapturous. I asked her what part of the house she would like to have and she said, 'I want to make the shop into a bed-sitting room for the two of us. Do it up for me, darling.' She was right, of course. The shop no longer looked like a shop but a bright sunny room with large windows overlooking the tree-lined drive and the rustic stone cow-sheds of the next-door farm. The room was big enough to combine a double bedroom with living room furniture so that visitors could feel that they were coming in to a small apartment rather than a sick-room.

When I returned home, I enlisted the help of Margaret, our cleaning woman, and between the two of us we transformed the shop into an attractive and functional bed-sitting room. As far as part-time help in nursing Jean was concerned, Vivienne had agreed to give up her job and be paid as companion-help; she and Edgar could live in the rest of the farmhouse rent-free and we decided to offer the cottage to our middle son, Clive, so that he could have the independence he craved. Jean was genuinely pleased over the arrangement with Vivienne for she saw this as an expeditious time to tutor her in the various arts of homemaking, something which had been a bone of contention in leading up to the marital rift. Once again, Jean saw herself as someone with a mission.

The moment when the ambulance brought Jean back from Oxford was a very moving one for us all. It was as though she had come back from the dead; none of us had ever expected to see her at home again. When the ambulance doors opened, she was propped up as usual, smiling and waving, girding herself for the uncomfortable transference from ambulance trolley to her bed, a feat which the drivers performed with great skill. Once inside, Jean refused to lie down, anxious to show that she could just as easily sit on the side of the bed. I could see that she was making an effort not to break down when she said, 'Fancy me coming back home! I never thought I'd be here again.' Clive spoke for us all when he said simply, 'Good to have you home, Mum.' We were all close to tears, sensing the momentousness of the occasion. Jean was quietly triumphant and deserved to be after such an arduous but nobly-endured struggle.

Once in bed, she assumed command of the situation by issuing a series of instructions about changing a picture, moving a flower pot, or shifting some of the furniture about. We were willing automata at her command. 'What's for dinner?' she demanded. 'I'm hungry,' and I knew by then that she had made a brilliant recovery.

From the day Jean arrived back in Chippenham, the family instinctively developed a routine of caring for her, rotating our sessions with Vivienne assuming the greatest number of hours. We had learned over the past year that even short periods of time can seem endless and one person cannot offer unlimited moral sustenance to a sick person. Interchangeability was necessary and we learned to rotate our nursing sessions to that the burden was never too cumbersome for any one person, including myself. We resumed the old routine of caring for her, reinforcing one another through our mutual efforts, sustained as always by Jean's persistent, quiet courage.

Within a few days, she had divined what she thought was the

means of being a well-dressed convalescent. Tired of nighties, housecoats, and drab hospital gear, she had scoured the newspapers and lighted on some advertisements in the *Guardian* for kaftans, striking long gowns which she thought would endow her sick-room role with the 'necessary elegance', as she quipped. She ordered two from Fenwicks of Bond Street, and insisted that I greet the postman in person at half past seven every morning so that we might not miss their arrival. The fact that Jean had ordered the gowns indicated to me that she was gearing her life to a slow but gradual recovery.

The ritual of anticipating the kaftans was like waiting for a long-expected Christmas present and, when the parcel did arrive, Jean was like a young girl with a party dress. I put the package on the bed and decided to leave the room so that she could try them on in peace; when I returned, she was standing somewhat shakily in front of the mirror assessing every conceivable angle of herself in the pink kaftan. She asked the typical question, 'Do you like it?' In fact, the gown became her and I told her so. She was tall and could carry off the style well and I made some comment about her bringing high fashion to Langley Burrell. Vivienne came in to have a look and they lapsed into a discussion of fashions, fads, and style in general, at which point I slipped out into the garden.

It was moments like this which gave us the brightest and happiest times. Jean was well relaxed; due to the quantities of drugs she was taking, she slept well at night although she could not move in the morning until she had taken her first dose of medicine. Actually we were administering massive doses of strong drugs which would normally be handled only by senior nursing staff in the hospital. To obviate any errors, we drew up a large chart based on instructions from Jean's doctor which indicated the type, amount, and time taken of the particular drug. Through painstaking efforts, we were able to look after her without fear of an overdose by accident. From the onset of the illness, Jean was given mild doses of tranquillizers to reduce any anxiety but the amount was nominal. At no point were anti-depressants administered.

The rapport between Vivienne and Jean was excellent and I could see a strong and sympathetic friendship in the making. It was asking a great deal for a seventeen-year-old girl to shoulder

66

the responsibility of a dying mother-in-law but she adapted to her duties admirably and Jean was extremely fond of her. We had been delighted to have three sons in our marriage but had regretted not having at least one girl and I could see that Vivienne was becoming for Jean the daughter she had never had. The bond between the two made looking after Jean that much easier and I began to return to my job in London whenever I could.

Jean's temperament was entirely stabilized by now and she kept in close touch with the world at large through other people's involvements. We learned to go to great lengths recreating even the most simple of our daily experiences for her. When Vivienne and I went to Cowidge Farm, buying glassware and bits of furniture, Jean was delighted when we brought her our acquisitions, describing in great detail the preview and the bidding at the auction. She showed no frustration over her lack of mobility but experienced vicarious pleasure from the actions of those closest to her.

One of her greatest pleasures was the masterminding of a speech which she had arranged for me to deliver to the Langley Burrell Women's Institute. She was responsible for booking me on a particular evening, having decided that it would be most edifying for the local ladies to hear about the world of Fleet Street. When I cried, 'What on earth have I got to say that's going to interest these countrywomen?' she produced a list of subjects which provided more than the bulk of my speech. 'Just tell them these things and then throw it open to questions. You'll be all right,' she declared breezily, and informed me that the highlight of my speech should centre around the evening I gave a special talk to the wrong audience in Manchester and the story for which I am most notorious – having reported six lions as being dead in a zoo fire only to discover later that they had miraculously survived the blaze ('the time Humphry killed six lions single-handed' as it is known).

The talk was in fact a grand success and I could only attribute this to Jean's planning and suggestions, not to mention her good memory. Instead of offering me the usual speaker's fee, the chairwoman asked if I would prefer to have a collection taken and the proceeds sent to the Imperial Cancer Research Fund. I thought this an excellent idea and admired the forthrightness of these countrywomen, all of whom were aware of Jean's condition.

67

For them, there was no shilly-shallying of finer feelings; cancer was something to be fought. When I arrived home and told Jean about the success of the speech and the collection taken, I could see that she was pleased. She settled down to sleep, well contented in the knowledge that she still had a sphere of influence in the outside world, however small.

Jean did insist, however, that she be provided with her own line of communication for people outside the family: I had the length of the lead on the telephone adjusted so that it reached her bedside, and she was able to keep in close touch with a fairly large circle of friends. She spent little time in bed, preferring to lie on top of the bedcovers in one of her kaftans, wearing short stockings and gold slippers. Because she rarely moved when visitors were present, thus not showing the severe limitations of bodily movements due to weakness and pain, outsiders thought she appeared to be extremely healthy. Her mind was always active; her interest in world affairs and local politics had never subsided and it was possible for someone not knowing the circumstances of her illness to speak with her and go away with the impression that there was virtually nothing wrong with her. Certainly they were incredulous on learning that Jean was in fact dying and was well aware of it.

It was this attitude which enabled Jean to survive, and, taking limited comfort from mundane things, she was content during these months. Only once did I catch her in a depression, when I discovered her morbidly contemplating the vast tray of drugs on the desk in the sick-room. I asked her what she was doing and she replied grimly, 'I've been wondering whether to end it all.' I could see she was depressed although I was not aware of anything that could have triggered it off. 'There's no need to talk like that, darling,' I told her. 'We have our agreement. Things are going well at the moment and let's concentrate on that.'

She returned to bed and resumed her normal activities never mentioning the incident again. Yet it gave me a fleeting glance of what was in the back of her mind. We did not talk about death. We had settled the matter and had no need to agonize over it. We were both people who knew our own minds as well as knowing and trusting one another. We had said enough in previous moments of crisis to know where we stood. This temporary depression was the only crack in Jean's otherwise good spirits.

What made both of us hopeful at the time was the fact that Jean was on a particular course of drugs – intensified hormone treatment – which the doctors said might well succeed in restraining the cancer. We clung to this possibility fiercely. Jean began to use her wheelchair more frequently and became quite competent in getting around the house. She would say, often quite gaily to anyone she happened to confront on her rounds, 'I'll be quite happy to settle for life like this – in a wheelchair – if only I can live.'

Yet in truth she was slowly declining. The facility for looking after herself thoroughly, together with her routine of moving about just so much, gave a false radiance to her appearance. This regimen and control made her appear less ill than she was, although I could see the subtle signs of deterioration. She was fooling herself and others as to the real state of her health but the deception provided us with a blissfully happy reprieve which lasted well into October.

7 BREAKDOWN

However, as we were to discover, trouble was never far away and, when it struck, it was a period which I can only think of as a descent into my own private hell. On the Monday following my talk at the Women's Institute, Jean collapsed in severe pain. Dr Gornall came immediately, intensified her sedation, and ordered that she be taken to the Oxford hospital as soon as possible. Her 'pain-spots' had erupted like a blitz and she needed radio-therapy badly to alleviate the acute discomfort. This turn for the worse signalled the end of another phase: the hormonal treatment which the dotors hoped would retard the cancer had obviously not done so and Jean was suffering badly.

Once again, she was transported by ambulance to Oxford and this time there was no doubt that she was absolutely comatose during the entire ride due to such excessive sedation. At least, I thought to myself, she is spared the agony of the ride and the anxiety of not knowing what lies ahead. Once again, I went through the ritual of driving to Oxford daily to see her, commuting either from Wiltshire or London, arriving at two in the afternoon, breaking for an hour at tea-time, and sitting with her until nine in the evening. I began to feel increasingly exhausted and my state of mind was not helped by the fact that Jean was rarely conscious during my visits. Often I would be with her for as long as six hours without a word or gesture being exchanged; I would merely sit in

71

silence, waiting for I knew not what, watching her drugged and unconscious.

To break the monotony, I changed my tactics and drove to London more frequently, staying with friends or at a small hotel close to the office. By keeping away from the farmhouse and being with other people more, I hoped to ward off a devastating depression which I could feel hovering over me. What fortified me was the patience, loyalty and hospitality of my friends. Perhaps these helped take the edge off the agony of my plight although I realized that no amount of good deeds could redeem me entirely from my own private hell.

Jean emerged slightly from her comatose state but this was by far her most gruesome relapse and we were both feeling pretty battered. In her occasional moments of consciousness, she was undoubtedly aware of the debilitating effect which her illnes was having on me. We were exhausted by the intermittent nature of the cancer, hitting us whenever we began to feel hopeful and had started to coast a bit. Our spirits were not elevated by the knowledge that this latest deterioration was accompanied by thrombosis in the legs, a condition not uncommon to cancer sufferers. Unfortunately, the thrombosis could not be treated because the medicine used to counteract it clashed with the cancer drugs. Thus Jean's legs began to swell badly and became extremely painful. Within ten days she was much worse and, once again, excessively drugged to prevent pain.

At this point, I knew enough to realize that I was on the way to a breakdown myself. Severe fatigue was my biggest problem and I noticed that I would fall asleep anywhere at any time as soon as I sat down. I dozed off in my car on the motorway to Oxford, awaking with a start to find myself overtaking another car at ninety miles per hour. Perhaps I only slept for seconds but I was frightened by this, pulled over into the lay-by, and fell asleep immediately. I was on the move all the time and I became plagued by the bemused feeling that I hardly knew where I lived or belonged. In fact, I was shifting about from one place to another with no regularity or security, whether at a colleague's house, a hotel, or the farmhouse in Wiltshire. My life became a complete chaos. There was only one reality for me the entire time: I was waiting for Jean to die, Yet, was this the time when she would in fact die, or would it lead to another spurious recovery followed by yet another relapse, always more painful and agonizing than the previous one? The end-of-the-year death sentence had already been foretold by the doctors and it was now almost November. I did not know what to believe.

I lived only from day to day, each moment revolving around Jean's pain and consciousness, and the ubiquitous fear of relapse, crisis, and death. This reaction became reflexive more than reflective. I continued doing stories for the newspaper in the hopes that the work would keep me preoccupied but I began to get facts wrong and I made some fairly serious mistakes. I felt professionally washed up in that I was simply no longer able to operate effectively. Mercifully, my colleagues were sensitive to my predicament and showed great tolerance and sympathy. Thus I continued working in a limited capacity in the hope that I could become occasionally involved in something other than Jean's illness. When I was not working, I found the hours heavy on my hands. Only people in a similar situation can have any idea how extraordinarily long the day and night can be. Driving back and forth to Oxford, fighting my way through traffic jams, visiting friends and colleagues became a way of killing time and, in a restricted sense, a mild form of therapy.

I realize now that everything in my life was rapidly being undone and taken away from me and as a result many of my moral values were ebbing away. There was a general feeling of my being endlessly hammered with the unpleasant aspects of life and the thought continued to persist in my mind that very little in my life mattered any more. Everything was topsy-turvy and I had to resist giving way entirely to a sense of imbalance. I was being torn in two different directions: preparing for life without Jean, which I knew was going to be terrifically difficult, and yet having to cope with a sick and ailing Jean, still alive and desperately needing me.

Certainly I had considered what life would be like after Jean was gone and I had to consider as well whatever contingencies might arise. Jean herself had spent a considerable amount of time talking to me and even counselling me about how I could best cope with my new life. In our own way we were preparing me for life ahead on my own. I resented other people's questions

73

about my future life but with Jean I could talk more openly and we would discuss what I would do with the farmhouse, how I could develop my career more, and even speculate about my remarrying. Given that she had been so close to death several times, I was steeling myself for life without her and was being pushed into it as much by Jean as anyone else.

In realizing that death was imminent and knowing how important the love for me was between man and woman, Jean put most emphasis on my need to remarry eventually. Due to her efforts more than anyone else's, I was trying to adjust to that possibility which would arise at some point in the next few years although I was not without deep fears and apprehensions. My anxiety was compounded by the fact that I was still very much in love with Jean, whom I wanted desperately, and did not wish to lose. Yet undoubtedly, part of me was exhausted by the entire struggle and I did not know quite which way to turn. There was no way I could resolve the conflict of having to cope with the present, to invest so much of myself in it, while trying to anticipate and plan for the future. My emotions took quite a battering, as I was clearly unable to integrate my feelings and sense of direction in any coherent way.

What impressed me more than anything was the fact that here I was, a man happily married for over twenty years, with three children, and suddenly, within less than a year, I was going to be a single man with no immediate family at all: Jean would be dead and the children were all getting married and drifting into lives of their own. It was highly confusing for a man accustomed to this wealth of security to find that, through no fault of his own, he is to be stripped of it. I realize that many middle-aged men long to be relieved of family responsibilities, yet most of them are afraid of the ultimate freedom because it is so terrifying in fact. But here I was, entirely against my will having this fantasy situation materialize through losing the one person who meant everything in the world to me and when the reality of remarriage confronted me – getting acquainted with, living with and loving another woman – I was riddled with anxiety and doubt over whether I could ever be attractive to another female. I hated thinking about all this and yet I could not resist it: everyone, including Jean, was coaxing me into realizing that life had to go on and for me this would have to include an involvement with another woman at some point in the future. For some inexplicable reason, the impact of this possibility hit me hardest when Jean was in the Oxford hospital. My moral reserves were depleted and I was frantic with exhaustion. It was during this time that I committed the only infidelity of my twenty-two years of marriage to Jean.

We had always been blessed with a marriage which was rewarding in many ways. We began life together when we were young and unpolished, inexperienced in the ways of the world and without any benefit of travel. Yet, as we progressed from a fairly simple way of life to a more sophisticated one, we were fortunate to grow together instead of apart, changing while generally complementing one another. Not least was the physical bond which continued to be strong and satisfying; there was never any need to turn to anyone else as Jean and I were genuinely happy with one another sexually even after we had been together for more than two decades.

In the initial stages of the cancer, there was no change in our sexual pattern and we continued as before. If anything, we were closer after the mastectomy for I realized how important it was to show Jean that the loss of a breast in no way made her less attractive so I believe that our bond was strengthened that much more. There was no change at all in our relationship until after our move to Wiltshire when the bone cancer started to erupt, causing a good deal of discomfort. As it became increasingly difficult for Jean to move with flexibility, sexual intercourse became more awkward. Gradually we came to realize that sex simply was not possible; it was quite painful for Jean and we both learned to generate our physical feelings for one another into an intense demonstrativeness. This was not easy for me but gradually I learned to accept it, seeing that I had no choice. By the beginning of 1974, we had ceased having any kind of sexual relationship. By the time Jean was in the hospital in Oxford, we had not made love for over ten months.

I think the imposed celibacy took more out of me than I realized at the time. It might have been easier coping with sexual frustration had Jean been absent; it seemed extremely difficult living with someone I loved, experiencing excessive affection for one another without at any time being able to consummate the love. Yet I knew Jean needed the affection badly and in many ways I needed it too. I indulged her with an abundance of love, sitting for hours holding her hand, often with both my arms around her. I could sense that she needed this attention in order to sustain her and in terms of touching and holding one another, we had never been closer.

However, the frustration began to wear me down physically and mentally. Jean, despite her illness, still looked very well. Visitors would ask me if in fact she were really as ill as they had heard because she was a striking woman who went to great lengths to keep herself looking as attractive as possible, even in the last stages of her illness. I still loved her intensely, undoubtedly more so now than I ever had, and to have her there yet so inaccessible was becoming more and more unendurable for me.

Certainly Jean was aware of how difficult the situation was and during the three months prior to her latest relapse she had discussed with me how awful it was to have had no love life for so long. She asked me outright if I would not be happier going to another woman to relieve the frustration and she said this on at least three occasions, emphasizing that she understood if I wanted to find someone else. However, I refused to discuss it with her as I thought it too preposterous. I did not want another woman, I wanted her, although I did not wish to say that to her as I was afraid it would only intensify her own guilt feelings. I just laughed it off in her presence and dismissed the whole subject as something that was not a problem, although undoubtedly it was.

I think that if Jean had not suggested the possibility that I relieve my sexual frustration with another woman, if she had not been preparing me for life with another woman in the future, I would not have committed the infidelity that I did. Without her suggestions, undoubtedly any involvement would have registered in my mind as a possibility to be experienced in the far future and thus pushed back into the inner recesses of my mind. Certainly I was not attracted by anyone else and the intensity of my affection was entirely monogamous. Yet it was Jean, to whom I had looked for so much my entire life, who in her own way had been preparing me to look beyond the two of us in other directions, to orientate myself in different ways. She was weaning me, of course, teaching me to rely less on her and to disengage myself from her guidance and stand on my own judgement. This must have taken immense courage on her part and caused considerable pain. The effect was to provoke in me the realization that I would eventually have to become involved with someone else and it was through Jean's tutelage that I was beginning to make the transition. Not that I had anticipated any involvement before Jean's death; the idea had simply never occurred to me. However, what I was doing was assessing myself more and more as an independent party with a new life to look to.

With Jean's latest relapse, I was again in the throes of a death-watch. Yet there was a finality about this one, perhaps because I was now the one who felt on my last legs as well. In desperation, I felt I had to turn to someone in an attempt to prove I could survive, if for nothing else. I knew that Jean was going to die and the prospect of being alone both shattered me and stimulated me into action. I was exhausted and terrified and I had to reach out to someone. It would have to be a woman. It was through a woman that I had had the most satisfying relationship of my life and so, almost without thinking, it was to a woman that I wanted to turn once again.

However, things were not that easy. Having had no sexual relationship with anyone other than Jean for over twenty years, I had little self-confidence. I felt isolated and uncertain. I doubted whether I was still attractive to women. I was nagged by the suspicion that I could never generate any enthusiasm on anyone else's part but I felt compelled to disprove my suspicion for I could no longer live with it.

Of course I had no idea where to begin my quest and, lacking any self-confidence, I decided it might be better to have sexual relations with a woman in an entirely impersonal setting. Some years earlier, I had done an article for my newspaper about an escort agency in Chelsea and I struck up a good rapport with the fellow who headed the outfit. I realized that I might be able to phone him and explain my problem and possibly he might have some bright ideas. I called him one evening after I had driven from Oxford to London; luckily, he remembered me and asked me to come round for a drink. I travelled to Chelsea and talked to him at some length in his office, explaining my circumstances and pouring out my problems to someone who was practically a complete stranger. He was very sympathetic and took me to a wine bar, buying a bottle of wine which we consumed pretty rapidly. During the evening, he said he knew a girl whom I might like and that I could go and visit her. After a few drinks, he telephoned her to make arrangements and, when he returned, he said I could go and see her within an hour, assuring me that we would have a very successful evening together.

I realized as I went to the girl's flat that she could be nothing more than a call-girl. Yet I was not in the least sobered by any sanctimonious feelings. I felt utterly devoid of moral scruples, and any conscience I had had simply ceased to function. I was motivated by a blind desire to survive regardless of the means. Morals had little to do with it.

I rang the bell at the girl's flat but was thrown into a dilemma as soon as she appeared. When I saw her, I knew that, despite whatever desperation I may have felt, there was no way I could work up any enthusiasm for her. She was fairly young and not unattractive, but there was a harshness about her which radiated in the most appalling manner. As I sat talking to her in her flat, I became even more convinced that I was an utter fool to be in a situation like this: I realized that I could never make love to a total stranger. I became increasingly uncomfortable as we continued talking about her Birmingham background and the few books which she had. I grew frantic trying to figure out some way of disentangling myself and I kept thinking to myself that this was no way to ease my frustrations. The escape clause presented itself when, lacking anything else to say, I asked her how much she charged for her services and she answered forty pounds. I hadn't the gall to tell her that I did not fancy her so mercifully I was able to deny having forty pounds on me, despite her willingness to accept a cheque with a banker's card. I denied having my cheque book with me and at this point things became very awkward. I got up to leave. She was offended and became uppity about my refusal. I was struck by the sordidness and implausibility of it all.

The incident with the call-girl had thrown me. I now considered that any encounter was fruitless and I began to give up hope of reaching out to anyone. I remained in London the following day, driving to Oxford that afternoon to see Jean, and when I returned to London that evening I made a dinner engagement on the spur of the moment with an old acquaintance whom I had known professionally for some time. She was female, and perhaps in the back of my mind I had an intuition of what might happen – but I can honestly say that in my conscious mind the date meant nothing more than a pleasant way to fill my leisure hours.

Undoubtedly I was feeling receptive to sympathy over my plight and probably asking for it in indirect ways. The evening turned out to be long and boozy and I found myself unfolding my problems to someone who, unlike my confessor of the previous evening was a warm and acutely understanding woman. Whether it was the wine and the gradual unfolding of my story which encouraged a sense of intimacy between us, I shall never be entirely certain. However, when we returned to her flat the chemistry was ignited and the inevitable happened. I like to think that I just gave way to all the pressures which had been building up for some time and I relinquished myself to whatever fate had in store for me. Needless to say, I was filled with a wealth of gratitude for this girl.

To be perfectly honest, the affair was immensely pleasurable and infinitely relieving. I remained with this girl for two successive nights, commuting to Oxford during the day and returning to her flat in the evening. She had met Jean some years before and was overwhelmed by the predicament of Jean's and my life together for the last two years. On the morning after the second night we spent together, she told me she simply could not continue with the affair under these circumstances; it was too unhealthy for everyone concerned and she was too intelligent and sensitive to tolerate the implications of the involvement. I did not blame her in the least for wanting to break it off. Originally she had acted more out of pity for me than anything else, but later came to realize that she could be hurt by our friendship. I sympathized with her point of view. Although I would have liked to continue seeing her for her companionship as much as anything else, I had too much respect for her to persist in a relationship in which she had everything to lose and nothing to gain. We put an end to our brief affair and I remember two distinct emotions as I left her flat and got in my car to drive to Oxford: one was reproach over the thought that I might have used this girl and hurt her by making her a vehicle for my own satisfaction; on the other hand I could not help feeling tremendously relieved over the fact that I could relate to another woman. All was not lost. I was capable of communicating with someone whom I considered attractive and she was capable of responding to me in turn. This knowledge did wonders for my ego and I no longer felt condemned to a life of utter desolation and solitude.

That very afternoon when I returned to Oxford I was confronted by the Sister on my way in to see Jean. She presented me with the good news that, wholly unexpectedly, Jean had started to respond to the recent combination of drugs administered and there was a good chance that she would recover from this particular relapse. The radio-therapy had suppressed the pain to the point where her body had begun to rally strength once again. The doctors now wanted to try chemotherapy on her as an additional treatment. We had accepted that the previous combination of drugs administered for the two months before the breakdown had failed. Chemotherapy was the last resort and could have some unpleasant side-effects but it could also cause the cancer to regress.

Jean was now conscious part of the time and the doctors approached both of us seeking permission to carry on with the chemotherapy. The treatment involved using drugs which were cellular poisons, killing tumourous cells in the body as well as some normal ones. Hair, gut, and bone marrow cells were those most radically affected; thus, baldness and severe indigestion were the possible undesirable side-effects and we had to discuss whether we wished to tolerate all the facets of the treatment. Despite the fact that Jean was excessively weak from her latest set-back, she was receptive to any course of medication since she was still hopeful of a cure. I remember her saying in the most determined manner, 'Well, I can always wear a wig if I lose all my hair and, what's more, get the National Health to pay for it all.' She was also encouraged by reports that chemotherapy induced greater mobility. I had noticed that the closer Jean came to death, the more she was prepared to fight. She had no illusions at this point over her close brush with death. She also realized that the chemotherapy would be the third and final treatment and there was no recourse to anything beyond that. Yet she was entirely philosophical about the hair loss and argued that no one was going to see her so appearances did not matter at a time like this.

The one thing she was adamant about was that she be allowed to return home. Family had always meant the world to her and without our presence at the farmhouse, she could not have endured so much. The consultants had encouraged her to return to Chippenham after the initial stages of the chemotherapy as they were all well aware of how important being at home was to Jean's peace of mind. They also realized what competent nurses we had all become and it was with their blessing that, once again, we prepared to bring her to Pinchloafe House.

In my diary, I have written on 28 October, 'Jean worsening', and it was during that week that her death seemed imminent. Yet, within ten days, she was at home again, looking somewhat weaker, but with as much spiritual resolve as ever. The ambulance men, by now well acquainted with the route between the farmhouse and the hospital, delivered her as they had many times before. We were all waiting for Jean in the drive, once again experiencing a feeling of incredulity that she was still with us. Yet I observed that we were all – including Jean – much more matter of fact about the homecoming as well as being definitely subdued. Obviously everyone was worn out by the ordeal. Although we were grateful to be together again, we were undoubtedly aware that we were graced with a reprieve which would be very short-lived. I could not help but steel myself for another relapse which I knew would be worse than the previous one, and I was aware that beneath the veneer of officiousness and stoic good cheer, Jean knew that this was her last homecoming.

I sensed a slight change in Jean although initially it was altogether subtle. It was on the evening of our second day at home that Jean,

81

once again, began talking about the fact that we had had no love life for so long, expressing her guilt over her own sense of failure. Had she guessed at what had happened? I remember her saying to me with utter directness that I simply must feel free to take another woman as a lover if I felt that it would make things more endurable for me. The conversation was so direct and spontaneous and Jean and I had always been so totally honest with one another that I replied, almost without thinking, 'Well, I have.' As simply as that. I could see instantly by the look on her face that I had made a dreadful mistake in admitting this to her and that, despite her pleas for me to relieve my frustration elsewhere, the knowledge that I had gone ahead and made love to another woman was a real blow. Realizing my mistake, my sense of loss was as dramatic as it had been in June when I had had to tell her that she was going to die. She looked at me, hesitating for a fraction of a second and said, almost inaudibly, 'Oh.' Nothing more. She was stunned and the dismay on both our parts was overwhelming.

In desperation, I insisted on talking about the encounter rather than have both of us fall silent with Jean supposing all kinds of things which had not happened. I thought to myself that, having gone this far, I should try and explain a bit more about the circumstances. Thus I filled her in with an abridged version of my brief encounter leaving out the incident with the call-girl. I apologized profusely and explained that it was due to a relapse on my own part, caused by the fact that I was desperate and exhausted and partly because she had insisted on my finding fulfilment if necessary. Jean agreed that she had encouraged this and she was not in the least reproachful although I could see that it was taking every bit of her courage and fortitude not to break down.

Without her asking, I promised that such a thing would not happen again and she acquiesced on this point. We tried to interpret the affair as a weakness under pressure and accept it as that. Eventually we kissed one another good-night and went to our separate beds although I noted how reflective she seemed. Before I went to sleep, I realized that a part of her had been trying desperately to make things easier for me by encouraging me to find some form of relief, but that, underneath it all, she had never wanted it to happen at all. With the infinite wisdom of hindsight, I wondered why I had not guessed this in the first place, saving her

82

such heartache. She was having to pay the price for her selflessness in the worst possible way and I found it difficult to sleep, speculating on what went through her mind that night.

When I awoke the next morning, I could see that Jean was already awake in the bed beside mine. I said good morning to her and started to get out of bed in order to prepare breakfast for the two of us. As I stood up, she turned to me and said very quietly, 'Come to bed with me, Derek, and make love to me.' I was overwhelmed by what she said and yet I was so longing to be with her that I approached her without saying a word and got into bed with her. Miraculously, the chemotherapy with which she had been treated for several weeks had promoted the resilience which the doctors had mentioned and Jean was blessed with a flexibility which she had not experienced for almost a year. We were able to make love happily and joyously as we had done for so long. Our loving was careful and restrained but infinitely satisfying to us both.

From that moment on, our sexual life returned to normal and continued until two weeks before her death. It was as good for her as it was for me. She was to live for four more months and during this time we lived as a sexually happy man and wife. The chemotherapy had worked a miracle in suppleness and made this reunion possible. We were terribly grateful for that. I like to think that some good came out of the thoughtless admission of my temporary infidelity which neither of us mentioned again. It seemed we were both determined to make the situation work for us. And we did.

8 DAYS OF GRACE

Once again, we resumed our former schedule with Jean and I living in the shop and Vivienne acting as nurse for Jean in my absence. Having had such an intensive training period administering medicine in the past, we were old hands at coping with the massive doses of drugs which were now necessary.

Chemotherapy produced a radical improvement in Jean. I could see that she looked a lot better and because of the physical change her spirits were unusually high. During this time our regular doctor from Chippenham, Dr Gornall, was away on holiday and I vividly recall the reaction of his deputy when he came for the routine weekly examination. After having spent the necessary twenty or thirty minutes with Jean, he walked down the drive with me to his car asking, 'Does she *really* know how ill she is?' in the most incredulous tone. I answered that yes, she did, and he went on to add, 'But does she know that the cancer has spread to other parts of her body?' Once again, I confirmed that nothing had been withheld from her. I remember, not without wry amusement, that he began to mutter more to himself than to me, 'How remarkable that she is like that, to answer all those questions so normally and cheerfully, to be so objective and, well, uh, *normal* really. What an extraordinary woman!' At this, he put his bag in the boot of the car, got into the driver's seat and, still muttering to himself, drove away.

However, notwithstanding Jean's good spirits, I always felt that disaster was right around the corner. I had arranged with the office to cover as many West Country stories as possible so that I could spend the maximum amount of time at home. I thought that this would keep me close to Jean while taking some of the edge off my own anxieties but this was not always the case, as there were the occasional cruel reminders of what fate held in store for me. I was researching a story on an ecological controversy concerning nearby Upton Cow Down in which there was a plan by a company to cut off an important hilltop in order to use the underlying chalk for commercial purposes. The removal would do irreparable harm to the landscape and I set out to interview some of the people living in nearby farms and villages to test their reactions to the plan.

The door of one farmhouse which I approached was answered by a lady of very sober manner and dress. She informed me that her brother owned the farm but she was uncertain whether he would be able to speak to me: his wife had just died of cancer and he was overcome with grief. As she said those words to me I felt panicky, realizing that this would be my situation in a matter of time and I wanted to flee from the spot. Mentally I had to rivet my feet to the front porch as I waited for her to return to tell me if her brother would grant me an interview. If she had not returned within a few seconds, I am certain that I would have run away. As it turned out, her brother did see me and I went through the ritual of asking him the necessary questions. By the end of the interview, I could see that he had been glad to see a new face, and was relieved to talk about something other than his wife's death but I was anxious to leave and concentrate on other things.

That afternoon I drove with the photographer covering the story to a spot where we could get a proper picture of the hill. His wife had accompanied him that day and while he crossed a field, angling for the right shot, she and I sat in the car waiting. In the midst of our small talk she mentioned that she had heard how ill my wife was and asked me if Jean were feeling any better. It was curious how I answered, 'No, she's dying of cancer and has very little time left.' She turned to me with an expression of utter incredulity and exclaimed, 'My God, how *do* you cope?' I did not find this question particularly overwhelming and I recall replying quite matter-of-factly, 'Well, you just do.' And that was that. If her question was not rhetorical, there was no real answer to it except the obvious: that there was no choice but to cope and one did without questioning the process. Surely this has something to do with the urge for survival and the ability to transcend one's difficulties although I have never been able to translate it into any definitive formula. It just struck me that neither Jean nor I had charted our survival course at the onslaught of the cancer. We merely behaved as two creatures following the instinct for keeping alive and it was a far more intuitive than cerebral process.

Nevertheless, some effort was necessary to keep us headed in the right direction. We had always valued a surface appearance of calm and normality and it was our ability to continue with daily life in this way that gave us the strength to persist. We also made a concerted effort to acknowledge that there was a future despite the fact that silently we realized we might not be sharing it together. Jean's concern for Vivienne and Edgar, the upkeep of the farmhouse, and the future developments in my career gave her a sense of purpose as well as the feeling that she still had a vocation in life. It was at this time that we made extravagant plans for the improvement of the gardens surrounding the farmhouse and cottage and we threw ourselves into the project with considerable enthusiasm. There were two acres of garden and orchard and we decided that after cutting back and pruning, a variety of fruit trees, shrubs and plants would provide the right balance. For several days, we sat in our room going through catalogues, making lists of our preferences. Eventually Jean drew up a final inventory and packed me off to a horticultural nursery in Bath with explicit instructions on what I was to purchase.

I returned several hours later with everything we had ordered spilling out of the back of the car and overflowing from the roof rack. I showed everything to Jean through the window seeking her approval and advice and it became gardening by proxy. 'Where do you want the cherry tree to go?' I would bellow, and she would direct me with, 'Down at the left-hand corner of the paddock,' and thus we would proceed. Through a series of shouted communications, exaggerated gestures, and dumb-show, we orchestrated the planning of the garden and orchard; in many ways we were like small children delighting in the prospects of how lovely it would

87

be in its fruition. Our extravagance was undoubtedly an expression of love for our home as well as for one another and an unspoken assertion of the need to accept the future and plan for it, with or without each other. I have no idea what was in Jean's most inner thoughts but I could feel her striving for the perfection which the grounds rightly deserved. Until the day she died, the garden remained an important focal point in her life.

During this time, Jean was returning to Swindon regularly for blood counts. The trips were relatively effortless due to the general improvement in her health and suppleness in her limbs, all of which could be directly attributable to the chemotherapy. She inspected her hair daily for fall-out but in fact it never happened; her hair was very fine and it stayed curiously intact until her death. The only unpleasant side-effect was some indigestion but whatever disadvantages Jean experienced were outweighed by her new-found agility, the main bonus of which was the ability to resume our love-making. This was such a blessing to us both that we found ourselves far more tolerant and mellowed towards life in general. The increased resilience gave Jean the mobility to take little walks around the ground floor of the house several times a day.

One crisp afternoon, I was working in the far end of the paddock clipping the apple trees in preparation for winter. This was a few days after Jean and I had completed our plans for the lay-out of the garden and only two weeks after she had returned from the Oxford hospital. As I was working, I had my back to the house and I thought I heard a voice in the distance. I realized that it was Vivienne calling to me to look around and, when I did turn, I could hardly believe what I saw standing at the foot of the paddock: it was Jean, fully dressed in her bright green slacks and brown leather coat, smiling at me with all the pride of her achievement. She had come to see the garden and she was looking to me for confirmation of the fact that this was nothing less than a miraculous appearance. And it was just that: here she was, having been so close to death so many times in the past, often unable to move because of excessive pain, not having been fully dressed for over a year, standing at the entrance to the paddock looking proud and happy. Neither of us spoke a word.

I could see that she probably had wanted to walk the full length of the garden but had been unable to and Vivienne, detecting that she could go no further, had called out to me. Finding Jean there, not twenty yards from me, was an uncanny emotional experience which threw me into a dazed silence. However, I realized within a few seconds that she was fully extended just standing there and must be exhausted by her efforts so I walked up to take her arm and steered her back in the direction of the house. As we walked, we talked about the wisdom of our planting and any changes we might make. Just before we reached the house, I released her arm and let her walk on her own with Vivienne at an arm's length, as I could sense that she wanted to demonstrate the extraordinary strength which remained with her. That small walk took a tremendous amount of effort but I knew she would feel it well worth it. I returned to the orchard and continued my work on the fruit trees, a very moved man.

Yet I felt ambivalent about the incident, nagged by the possibility of hope. Was this an indication that the chemotherapy, our last resort, *was* in fact causing the cancer to regress? Or was it only providing us with more spurious hope? Despite the overwhelming odds against us and the traumas we had experienced, one still hoped for the miracle to occur. Jean obviously thought that there was a possibility of recovery and without her saying, I could see that she was banking everything she had on it as well.

December proceeded fairly normally although the nursing of Jean became more difficult. There were even more drugs to administer and we had to stay a lot closer to her for she craved company and seemed to need more people around her than before. She never referred to dying during this period nor did she mention any possibility of my remarrying; all her conversations centred around the living. The chemotherapy continued to have a dramatic effect on her. Her iron self-discipline in forcing herself to get out of bed several times a day was the key to her therapy and sense of progress; she had no intention of ever being bed-ridden. She nursed a great deal of hope for recovery and I could see that she thought a regression of the cancer entirely plausible.

Despite signs of progress made possible by the new drug

treatment, I could observe tell-tale symptoms indicating that her condition was deteriorating simultaneously. Jean was gradually pacing herself down and this was due more to illness than uncomfortable side-effects such as acute indigestion or increasing overweight due to hormone treatment and inactivity. To the casual observer, she never appeared to be fighting the cancer yet I could see how she had developed a technique of moving and exerting herself only at the exact moment when she knew that the drugs would have their maximum effect. She would sleep all afternoon and long hours in the evening, taking pills immediately upon waking; she would keep very still and move only when the drugs began to have a heightened effect inhibiting the pain. I was anxious to prevent her from moving a great deal because I was aware that as the cancerous tumours replace the bone marrow, the bones become increasingly brittle and snap with the minimum of pressure. I could never lose sight of the fact that Jean was still a very sick person.

However, because Jean honestly thought she was on the mend, we started a ritual which was enacted every Wednesday morning when it was time for me to return to work. She would put on her very best face and assure me that she was feeling very well and had no need for my presence; she would urge me to go to London and continue with my regular working schedule there. She would say, typically, 'Do you have all your clean shirts to take with you and are your trousers pressed? I really *do* feel well, so don't worry about me.' Yet invariably I would phone Vivienne from London that evening and learn that Jean was worse. Not wanting her to suffer under those conditions, I would drive back that night or the following morning. It became a frequent routine: driving to London on Wednesday morning, ringing home that evening and discovering that she was worse, turning around and driving the one hundred miles back home within a few hours.

Vivienne coped very well with the situation but I could not stand being away from Jean under those circumstances. Often I would arrive at home and she would be so heavily drugged that it was some time before she became aware of my presence. When she did wake up, I would fabricate stories about there being nothing to do at the office or create an article that had to be researched in nearby Bristol, or even claim that there had been a strike at the

Times offices in London. Of course my excuses became transparent to her keen eye and one day she said very pointedly to me, 'I really think that we should sell the farmhouse and move back to London. I can see it's too much for you travelling back and forth and we want to be together without quite so much trouble for you.' I appreciated her thoughtfulness although I was also sorry that I had not fooled her entirely; I did not want her to feel guilty over being any kind of inconvenience to me. Certainly I was thunderstruck over the possibility of moving after all we had been through. I reassured her that I did not mind the commuting and that she was not to worry. I also reminded her that the real estate market was so utterly depressed at that time that we would have to stay right where we were but I also emphasized how much we loved the farmhouse and looked forward to a lovely Christmas which was only a few weeks away.

Before our Christmas celebration in Wiltshire, the office was planning their party at an Italian restaurant in Soho on the Tuesday night of 10 December. I did not relish the idea of going but Jean pressured me to travel to London as she always did. Once again, I could see that she was gauging her 'recovery' on the extent to which we were able to resume our old routine. The more I assumed a full and active schedule, the more reassured she felt that things were reverting back to normal. I realized it was a kind of a game in which I was the central player but my strategy had such a crucial effect on Jean's spirit that I simply had no other choice than to play along with the whole thing.

I drove to London and went to the party but made no attempt to stay sober or even responsible, wallowing instead in a very drunken evening. Quite a few of us continued the party at the flat of one of our female reporters. Despite the fact that I had a lot to drink, I recall a discussion with another journalist from our paper who was an avid diarist. He knew about Jean's illness and kept insisting on how important it was to record on tape as many of my conversations with Jean as possible. I found the idea dreadfully offensive and told him so although I did not explain why. Inwardly, I realized that this kind of behaviour would have brought me closer to signing Jean's death warrant – especially in Jean's eyes – and it was the kind of gesture of finality that neither she nor I wanted any part of. Recording death-bed conversations would have appalled her, robbing her of any illusions of recovery.

I was able to return home the following day except that in this instance it was due to my own deterioration and not Jean's. I had passed out on the living room floor of the flat at four in the morning but had only slept an hour in all. I got up at the crack of dawn with a mammoth hangover and depressing thoughts. Somewhat frantic for something to preoccupy me, I started to clean the kitchen and living room, becoming so excessive in my zeal that I vacuumed and mopped floors as well as washing up dishes and glasses and putting out bottles and garbage. I phoned Jean after I had had breakfast to tell her I would be returning to Chippenham although I did not want to reveal to her the real reasons for my misery. I rarely had hangovers because I seldom had more than a few drinks; if she realized how much liquor I had consumed the night before, she would suspect that things were bothering me far more than I let on. I merely told her that I was coming down with a cold and would be home within a few hours. I noticed how weak her voice was on the phone despite her efforts to convince me that she was feeling fine and I could detect a sense of decline one hundred miles away. I knew that she very much wanted me to be with her.

Christmas could not have come for us at a better time. Jean's struggles to appear normal were taking their toll and she needed the diversion of some activity other than her illness. She had admitted to me at one point that this might be her last Christmas but when she said this to me there was no defeatism in her tone; instead it was predicated by the comment that she was determined to make it the best celebration ever. In her waking hours, she made several long and elaborate shopping lists, revising each list several times. Finally, she sent Vivienne and I to Bath with instructions on where to purchase everything and how much we should spend. If something was not exactly what she wanted, she would send us back to exchange it and in one instance we had to return to Bath three times! However, we did not mind in the least, as her involvement in the Christmas project was so salutary that we all became quite infected with her enthusiasm.

Jean was determined to have a full house on Christmas day and she inveigled Vivienne – not an enthusiastic cook – into making preparations for an enormous Christmas feast, helped by Aunt Stella from Bournemouth. Jean wrote to Godson asking him to join us and she sent invitations to friends and neighbours in the area to call in for a Christmas drink. When Christmas day arrived, Jean awoke even earlier than usual and spent a good deal of time arranging her hair, making up her face, and putting on a special rose-coloured kaftan. It never ceased to amaze me how her spirits were capable of swinging into such full and positive gear. We exchanged presents in the living room at eleven o'clock that morning and Jean walked with only the aid of a walking stick through the breakfast room, along the twenty-foot kitchen and up the stone-slabbed corridor. Dinner followed the gift-giving and she remained throughout the first course after which she returned to her bed to finish her dinner there. Sitting upright was too uncomfortable for her and any change from a supine posture could only be endured for short periods of time. However, she spent the entire afternoon receiving callers in her room and playing the good hostess. We all remember it as one of the happiest Christmases we ever had as a family. None of us was depressed by the fact that this was undoubtedly the last we would spend with Jean. Her live-for-today philosophy had proven itself to be contagious and we learned from her to make the most of the moments we had together.

This peaceful interlude at home paid off for me professionally as well. In the past, I had tried to keep up with duties in the news room but my sporadic appearances in the office, my difficulty in keeping appointments, and my inability to concentrate had impaired my capabilities as an accurate reporter. The news editor agreed that it would be more useful and timely for me to conduct a long-term investigation into street crime in London, and this kind of story meant that I could work whenever it would be convenient for me. During more tranquil moments, I would drive to London and spend hours in the ghettoes, talking to youth workers, social workers, local politicians, and many members of the black community. It was my objective to determine precisely how serious street crime was in the inner city and whether black youngsters were the main perpetrators as had been alleged by many and, if so, why.

93

This method of working became extremely useful to me. I did most of my research the month before Christmas and it was during the week following Christmas that I sat down and began to write. It became one of the best pieces of journalism I had written in my thirty years of reporting and I could only attribute its success to the peace and calm with which we had been blessed in the preceeding weeks. The article had a wide impact and the fact that I had finally done something worthwhile was a real boost to both Jean and me, not least to myself for I realized that I still had my touch, something which I had begun to suspect might be gone forever. For days after the article appeared, the phone never stopped ringing and I was busy scheduling appearances on radio and television.

It was at that time that the publishers of my book on Michael X were inquiring about when I would be able to produce something, for work on the manuscript was a long way behind schedule. To date, both they and my co-author had been very understanding but the delay was becoming unreasonable and I realized that either I had to get started or pull out of the project altogether. I knew that the book would require a great deal of time and effort, things I had not much of at this point but, on the other hand, I could not afford to withdraw. During Jean's illness, my earnings as a free-lance writer had dropped from approximately one thousand pounds a year to nothing. A few months previously, I had cancelled a contract with Gollancz, the London publishers, for a book about the investigation of jury behaviour in British courtrooms and had had to return their three hundred pound advance.

Because Jean and I were so encouraged by the success of my article on street crime, we decided that I should continue with my plans for the Michael X biography. By January things were going better and Jean had no relapses or declines. I made plans to rent a flat in London with my co-author; my nomadic life had proved itself to be so unproductive that I thought if I were to live half the week in Chippenham and the other half in London working, the results might be fruitful. I was not certain that it would in fact work out that neatly but I knew that it was important to go through the acting-out of commitment and planning ahead, knowing that this was the one strategy which had the most beneficial effect on Jean's spirits.

Jean became very enthusiastic about the book and my move into the London flat. She began to organize my transfer, specifying which sets of sheets, blankets, and towels should be taken with me. Once again she was setting up a new home by proxy. She even said to me at one point, 'You know, when you get settled I'm going to come up to London and spend some time with you there.' I could see that her intentions were genuine and I found her determination, as always, poignant. I had learned not to contradict her although I did slip up on one occasion by mentioning that the iron spiral staircase leading to the bedroom and bathroom would be a difficult manoeuvre for her. She shot at me like a flash that I should not put obstacles in her way: 'I *can* get over things like that,' she huffed, and I could see that the subject was closed.

She wanted to play as active a part as possible in the preparation of the book so I made good use of her willingness by having her organize the scores of newspaper articles about Michael X. She performed the task in the most painstaking way, arranging every cutting in chronological order before putting them in the scrapbook. Her efforts saved me hours of tedious work. I think she began to feel that she was really pulling her own weight through her attempts to help me out and when she heard that we were now receiving a permanent disability allowance from the Department of Social Security, she was overjoyed. The money would pay Vivienne's wages and she realized that she might even be an asset to the family economy. 'Well, no one can say that I'm a drag on the finances now,' she commented and I could see that she said this with a considerable element of pride.

As they say, hope springs eternal and in looking back, I can see that this was precisely the feeling that had overtaken Jean and even myself to a point. By the time February had arrived, I had pushed into the back of my mind the fact that she was going to die. Indeed I was jolted back to reality when talking with an acquaintance in London about her health. 'I don't think I have ever met anyone in your situation who is waiting for their wife to die,' he said. I was flabbergasted by his words, not so much for their directness but because a part of me had ceased to acknowledge the situation as being just that. Undoubtedly I had been lulled into thinking that this period of grace might extend itself indefinitely.

Jean herself was guilty of encouraging this attitude. During February, we had arranged to have building contractors put a new stone-tiled roof on the cottage adjoining the farmhouse. Jean had complained that she could not see any of the work going on despite a running commentary from every member of the family on its progress. On the day the workmen finished, Jean could contain herself no longer. She got up and dressed herself with the aid of Vivienne, the second time she had done this in four months. The three of us went into the garden to inspect the cottage and she was delighted with the roof's appearance and the dormer window I had installed. After we returned to the farmhouse and she got back into bed, it began to snow and I commented on how nice it was that the cottage was better protected. Jean turned to me and said, 'You know, I'm glad we had it done. It will be such a lovely house for the future.' I was struck by her use of the word 'we', as well as by her thoughts for the long-term future. We had reached a stage where, on both our parts, the slightest inflection or particular choice of words carried every significance. She saw the future as including herself in some capacity. She felt that she might be here to share it with us for some time.

It was at this point that our adopted son Stephen, now eighteen, felt the desire to see his natural mother and I noted how philosophical Jean was over the whole affair. Two years earlier, when in the throes of an identity crisis, he had responded quite eagerly to my suggestion that he visit his mother whom I knew still lived in Manchester. However, after I had arranged a meeting through the Manchester adoption authorities, Stephen had backed off and never mentioned a reunion again until this particular time. Whether it was the prospect of Jean's death or a deep-seated resurgence of the perfectly natural desire to meet his real mother, neither Jean nor I were certain, but we willingly gave him our blessing to meet the woman who had given birth to him.

After the reunion took place, Stephen telephoned us to describe the experience and get additional reassurance from me that it was all right to go ahead and establish a closer rapport with his mother and the several brothers and sisters whom he had discovered. Ultimately he settled in Manchester to remain near them (and is still living there today). I found Jean's reaction enigmatic in a way; I felt that she could not help but be slightly hurt at the transfer of affection from one mother to another at such a crucial time. However, she only expressed her best wishes for Stephen, emphasizing how important it was for him to capture a sense of identity which had always escaped him. As she wrote in a letter to her father, 'Steve is going to see his Mum and brothers and sisters this weekend . . . as I said to him, he has the best of both worlds – two families!'

I began to suspect that Jean felt that there was plenty of time for her to re-establish contact with Stephen in the near future and, if she did nurture this belief, I was all too happy to encourage it. However, I could not help but contemplate how this was just another in a series of disintegrations of our once firmly intact family unit.

Our reprieve continued until one morning in the second week of March. Jean and I awoke as usual and I went to fetch a basin of water for her to wash, leaving it and the bathing materials on the table beside her bed. I went to sit on the sofa on the other side of the room to peruse the morning papers. Just as I began to read, there was a loud clanging noise; I looked around and saw Jean clutching for the bowl of water as it fell off the bed. She reeled back, grabbing at her ribs in what was obviously great pain and I ran over to assist her, picking up the scattered articles on the floor. She was gasping with discomfort so I hurried to phone the family doctor who said he would come over right away.

His diagnosis was what I had feared for months: one of Jean's ribs had snapped and the fact that this breakage was caused merely by bending forward too rapidly was the fatal signal. I knew that the effects of the bone cancer in its last stages were now emerging; if her ribs had broken that easily, it meant that any of her other bones could snap in an instant with minimal pressure. I asked the doctor about this and he confirmed that there was severe risk of other fractures.

Jean had no idea that this was a danger signal and adopted quite a cavalier attitude to the accident. She laughed as she remarked, 'Don't worry about me. As I'm in bed all the time, there'll be no problem in the rib mending.' However, I knew that the time had come to try and secure the drug which she could take to end her life. I knew from everything the doctors told me that it would be a struggle from now on.

When the Wednesday came and Jean applied the usual pressure for me to go to London, I did not resist as I knew it would give me the opportunity to see a physician about solving the dilemma of how Jean's life would end. I had not forgotten our pact made ten months earlier and I had no intention of letting her down. Intuitively, I knew she would be asking the question about death very soon.

I had not seen the physician from whom I was going to seek advice for some time and he did not know about Jean's illness. However, we had developed such a good understanding in our ten years' acquaintance that I knew he would grant me any favour I requested. I did not want to involve either of Jean's doctors in Wiltshire or Oxford; I did not know them well enough to confide in them and I could not help but feel that to involve them in a suicide pact was incongruous after they had worked so hard at prolonging Jean's life in the best possible way. I realized how fortunate I was to know someone else in the medical profession in whom I had unqualified trust.

I phoned my friend and made arrangements to see him at his Harley Street office that evening. When I told him the details of Jean's illness, he told me that certainly she only had a few weeks of life left. Further breakage of her bones was highly probable; bones in her legs could snap if she tried to walk just a few feet. 'I doubt if there is any decent existence left for her,' he said to me, 'and I wouldn't blame you in the least if you want to save her a great deal of pain and anguish.' I was overcome with gratitude for this man's sensibilities. He gave me a powerful combination of sleeping pills and pain-killers which would easily dissolve in water. He warned me that the bitter taste would preclude me giving the mixture to Jean without her realizing what it was. I thanked him for his help, we shook hands and he wished me well, and I prepared to drive back to Langley Burrell.

It seemed to me then that Jean was living on two planes. On one level – her outward mien – everything was going to be fine. She was going to live. An indication of this attitude is contained in a letter to her father written sixteen days before her death:

I have had a pain in my chest and at first the specialist couldn't find out what it was. Well, last week they did more X rays and, believe it or not, I've got a cracked rib. I think I must have done it when one of the bedside tables fell over with a bowl of water on it and I attempted to save the bowl from spilling. Anyway, they may take me into Swindon hospital and give me one of those pain-killing injections like I had in my spine. It's maddening just when I was managing to get out in the car, but on the other hand it could have been worse and at least this will soon heal up.

All this optimism while a part of her knew that the end was approaching. Yet she chose to compartmentalize this in a more remote corner of her mind – for the time being, anyway.

9 DECISIONS

A fortnight passed after the breaking of Jean's rib. Just after my return to Chippenham, I took all the pills and decided that it would be best to mix them into a liquid form ready to be administered at a moment's notice. I realized that when the time came to give them to Jean I would have to act quickly. Dissolving all the tablets into a thick brew, I hid the mixture in a room to which Jean had no access. From that moment on, I spent virtually all my time in the sick-room looking after Jean as painstakingly as I could. She was not in any alarming discomfort but it was obvious to me that she was becoming a relic of her previous self and slowly ebbing away. The tension for both of us was constraining and we worked very hard at not showing it to one another. We would sit together all our waking hours holding hands; I would often have my arms around her and we would listen to music. While she slept, the garden continued to offer me relaxation in the midst of the death-watch. Without the spells of fresh air and physical activity, I would have found my vigil intolerable. Jean was acutely aware of its healthy effect on me and she would always say to me when she felt tired, 'I'm going to sleep now, darling, you go into the garden.'

The only indication I had that Jean was contemplating putting an end to her own life occurred when Vivienne came in late one afternoon with two black kittens she had adopted from a nearby farm. She put them on the bed and they promptly began playing with Jean's bedclothes. As I came into the room, I could see the look of delight on Jean's face as she watched the two small creatures and she looked up at me, her eyes filled with tears, and said, 'Life really *is* worth living, isn't it?' She was such an unsentimental person, particularly about animals, that I could not help thinking to myself that she had a very clear idea how close she was to the end. She must have sensed that she would soon have to ask me the inevitable question about the carrying out of our pact. That she would have to surrender within a short time to death caused her to recoil in appreciation of the simpler dramas of life and this showed for just an instant with her over-reaction to the kittens.

At the end of a fortnight, I had to go to London quite suddenly to finalize arrangements for the printing of a little book, *The Cricket Conspiracy*, which I had written for the National Council for Civil Liberties. My departure would mean that Jean would be on her own for a twenty-four hour period and I was extremely apprehensive about leaving her without informing Vivienne of the existence of the overdose which I kept hidden. Obviously I saw myself in the role of compassionate executioner and I dreaded the possibility that Jean might break more bones in my absence and experience agonizing pain which should not have to be endured. The only alternative left to me was to tell Vivienne about the presence and purpose of the pills and, without instructing her to administer them necessarily in case of a crisis, I gave her the option to do as she pleased. Mercifully, she said she agreed with me and that if the situation became catastrophic, she would take the initiative and administer the overdose herself. Vivienne's equanimity provided me with more than a little solace although I could not help feeling as if I were holding my breath the entire time I was away.

As I had suspected, storm clouds were gathering. When I phoned home the following morning, I received the worst possible news. Vivienne told me that Jean had had intense pain in her neck all night; the doctor had been called and arrangements had been made for her to be taken to the Swindon hospital at midday to see her Oxford consultant who happened to be there. Jean would not be arriving until 2 P.M. so I decided to wait a few hours before driving the seventy-five miles to Swindon to meet her there. I knew then that the death-warrant was sealed. Jean had always said that when the cancer reached her neck, this would signal the end, for by then the disease would be close to the brain. Not to mention the fact that this new outbreak of pain meant that the chemotherapy which had worked so well for the past five months had now run its course; our last resort had failed. I walked aimlessly along Doughty Street, passing Charles Dickens's home, engrossed in my thoughts, killing the few intervening hours before I would drive to Swindon. Precisely how would I cope with Jean's end now that it was here? Frantically deliberating, I happened to run into a colleague and I recall answering his questions in absolute gibberish, completely unable to tune into anything he was saying. He gaped at me as if I were some kind of simpleton. Indifferent to him, I simply walked away.

When I arrived at the hospital, I found Jean lying on a stretcher outside her consultant's room. We kissed hello and I noticed how she tried to be as gay as possible under the circumstances making cheerful remarks to me and the nurses as they passed by. Typically, she gave no sign of capitulating. The crisis was approaching and she must have sensed this, yet her self-control was never more unwavering.

After the X rays had been taken, the consultant explained to us that there had been another outbreak of cancer at the top of the spine. He did not refer to the failure of the chemotherapy but this was implicit in his comments and I manouevred an opportunity to speak to him alone a few minutes later. 'What, if anything, can be done now?' I asked him. 'Is there any point in her going back into hospital now?' He confirmed my worst suspicions when he answered, 'We can relieve the pain to a certain degree but there is always the question of quality of life. She is worn out from fighting.' (Later Dr Laing told me that he had sensed at the time that Jean had given up. 'She didn't say so in words but she made it perfectly clear to me that she didn't want to prolong her life,' he said.)

I felt I did not need to ask him anything further. This latest attack was the last blow for Jean from which only death would provide the release. Since she had steadfastly refused to die in the hospital and had indicated this months before, I made arrangements for her to be taken back to Langley Burrell by ambulance and I followed in the car.

The next day was Good Friday and we passed it quietly in the sick-room. Although heavily drugged, Jean was awake for several hours at a time and during these hours she was alert and relatively cheerful. We merely lived out the day saying nothing special to one another, keeping whatever private thoughts we had to ourselves. It may seem strange that we said so little on that Friday which turned out to be our last full day together; however, when you have had to live with the possibility of death for as long as we had and it has dominated you in every way, you resist its grip particularly at the end, making every effort to keep whatever time remains to you exclusively yours. We sat quietly holding one another, listening to our stereo and occasionally reading. That evening I sat by her bedside and we played Jean's favourite pieces by Grieg as well as Franck's Symphony in D which we had seen performed on our first date together in Manchester in 1953. On our honeymoon we had visited Cesar Franck's home on the Left Bank in Paris and we reminisced about our wonderful trip. With effort, I tried to keep a hold on my emotions until Jean fell into a drugged sleep.

I knew that the end was imminent and I debated whether I should slip the overdose to Jean that night. I wanted so desperately to save her from the anguish which I knew she was silently enduring but I realized that I could not administer it without her knowing. Despite the fact that the cancer had been dissipating her body for two years and four months, I knew that she could live perhaps another three or four agonizing weeks while the disease ran its final savage course. I was solely concerned with Jean's well-being and I turned over the options of how best to carry out our pact and protect her from an horrendous end. I thought how nice it would be to give her something pleasant to drink and have her fade away quietly at a time when we were so happy.

For most of the night I turned this over in my mind until, exhausted, I fell asleep at dawn. What I did not know was that earlier in the afternoon, when I thought Jean was asleep and I had slipped into the garden, she had summoned the children individually and spoken about the way she would like things to be after her death. Not the least of her requests was that they do their

104

best to help me build a new life of my own. Jean had thought it all out and had spent the night preparing herself for death the following day.

10 'IS THIS THE DAY?'

When I awoke the next morning, I turned my head on my pillow and saw Jean was gazing at me. I sensed that she had been lying there looking at me for some time, waiting for the end of my sleep, and I was filled with the premonition that something was the matter. However, I said nothing apart from the usual, 'Good morning, darling. How are you feeling?'

'My neck is very bad. I can't move it,' Jean replied.

I climbed out of bed and prepared her usual dosage of medicines and pain-killing drugs which she swallowed in a gulp. I opened the curtains, remarking on what a clear and bright spring day it was but there was no reaction from Jean who was quiet and reflective, absorbed in her thoughts.

'Shall I get breakfast now?' I asked.

'Yes, good,' she replied. 'Just tea and toast.'

I picked up the morning papers on my way to the kitchen and began to prepare the snack. I kept thinking to myself, what shall I do if she asks if she has reached the end? Am I absolutely certain that it is close to the end? This was the one time when I could not fail her: I would have to be honest and say 'Yes'. I realized that the end was here for I had been seriously considering taking her life myself. She could not go on suffering like this any longer, particularly with the risk of more bone fractures which would mean

107

rushing her to the hospital to die there – something she did not want at any cost. I realized that, were she to go to the hospital on the following Tuesday for more radio-therapy treatment, she would never return home either. (Dr Laing told me later that immediately after he saw Jean for the last time in Swindon, he wrote to Dr Gornall in Chippenham: 'I am not anxious to prolong this woman's life at this stage. Nevertheless, one must do one's utmost to control the symptoms.')

I recalled Jean's words spoken a few months previously: 'When I die, I want to be at home with you, Derek, and only you and me. Whatever you do, don't let me die in hospital.' My eyes filled with tears and burned so much I had to bathe them in cold water. Trying to appear normal, I carried the breakfast tray into the sick-room, tossing the *Guardian* in the usual manner on to Jean's bed. For once she ignored it, preferring to sip her tea and nibble at her toast, looking out the window at the rose bushes. We were each buried deeply in our own thoughts. I was so tense I could not bear looking at her and kept my gaze directed towards the golden privet bushes lining the drive.

'Derek?' Jean called softly.

'Yes, darling.'

'Is this the day?'

I panicked. My mouth dried up and I could not control the tears which rushed to my eyes. It was the most awful moment of my life. However, I had to answer, 'Yes, my darling, it is.'

There followed many minutes of silence as we both considered the decision we had taken. Had I done the right thing? Was it too soon? Should she go back to the hospital for more treatment? My tormented thoughts were checked in the midst of their chaotic rambling by Jean's calm, measured voice. 'How shall it be? You promised me you would get me something.'

'I have,' I answered. 'A doctor in London has mixed me a combination of drugs which are quite lethal. You have only to take them and that is the end.'

We became silent again and I asked myself if I should cross-examine her about the correctness of her part of the decision. However, I resisted this because it was so apparent that she was depending on me for judgement. To raise any doubts at this point would only muddle the certainty and clarity of our instincts and intelligence. We both knew intuitively that this was the right time. To waver would have been wrong.

Again she spoke first. 'I shall die at one o'clock. You must give me the overdose and then go into the garden and not return for an hour. We'll say our last good-bye here but I don't want you to actually see me die.'

Nonplussed by her coolness, I could not help but agree with her. Jean resumed her breakfast, even glancing at the newspaper although she threw it aside after a few seconds. I realized how trivial the affairs of the world seemed when there were only a few hours left between us. Any indecision I had previously felt vanished now that Jean had confirmed the decision and chosen the time of her death.

I felt a massive load lifted off my mind knowing that I would not have to perform a mercy-killing on my own. Somewhat dizzy from the momentousness and drama of the situation, I exalted in Jean's courage, and sheer efficiency in carrying out her chosen way of death. After more than two years of suffering she was, I felt, entitled to leave this life with style and entirely on her own terms.

'Would you like a bowl of water, beloved?' I asked. She accepted it in the customary manner, washing her face and hands, brushing her teeth, combing her hair and applying a light lipstick. Afterwards, with my help, we straightened her bed. However, as we did this, the fierce pains shot through her neck and hastily I passed her more pain-killers. When they began to take effect and had suppressed the pain, she wanted to talk again.

'I'm so glad it has all been decided,' she said. 'It's a load off my mind.'

However, this reminder of the finality of it all after twenty-one full and happy years together – our anniversary was the following month – undid my self-control and I collapsed in Jean's arms, sobbing.

'You mustn't cry,' she murmured. 'After all, you're the winner in all this. You're young enough to go on again. You'll find some other woman to love. There are lots of women in the world who need a husband.'

'But I don't want to lose you,' I replied through my tears. 'Please don't leave me.'

'It can't be otherwise, darling,' she said, almost coolly. 'I've got this bloody cancer and I simply can't fight it any longer. But you must make a new life for yourself or else all that you and I have done together will be wasted.'

She implored me to stop crying and gradually I managed to get control of myself. We talked of our life together, the births of Edgar and Clive, the adoption of Stephen. We reviewed all the happy holidays we had spent in seaside cottages in Wales and Devon, camping holidays in France and Germany, and generally a life of love and devotion to the children and each other.

'I've only ever loved you, Jeannie,' I told her. 'I've never been unfaithful apart from that episode last autumn. And that wasn't love – it was a relapse due to strains which I simply couldn't bear. It was an awful lapse and I can only ask for your forgiveness.'

'If that was the only occasion in twenty-two years, then we haven't done too badly,' she said. 'We've put that behind us so don't let's talk about it now.'

When she asked me once again what I intended to do with Pinch-loafe House I recalled that it was the same day, Easter Saturday, two years earlier, that we had impetuously bought the farmhouse. I told her I would keep it for the time being and perhaps eventually arrange to sell it to the children.

'Yes, I'd like that,' she said. 'I'm so glad we moved here for the end of my life. It's made it much more bearable.'

She did not want to see anyone other than me that morning but when I left the room I took the opportunity to tell the children that I thought Jean was dying. They took it stoically so they must have sensed it earlier. No one suggested we call the doctor. At that time, I did not know that Jean had spoken to them the day before, giving them her last instructions and obviously saying good-bye to them at that time. When I returned to the room, Jean was sorting out the drawer in her bedside table. She threw away an empty compact, some old sweets, and cleaned off the table with a tissue.

'When I'm dead,' she announced, 'take off my rings. They always steal them in the crematorium. And give my clothes to my cousin and aunt in Manchester – they can keep what they want and sell the rest. And don't forget it's a holiday on Monday and you won't be able to register my death until Tuesday. And I don't need to make a will, I've got nothing to leave.'

A naughty smile crossed her face as she made the last remark.

110

She had always made wry comments about families who quarrel over wills and estates and it pleased her to leave the world poor but happy.

'There's one thing I want you to promise me,' she continued. 'You must go to Manchester after I'm dead and tell my father exactly how I died. I don't want him to think I died in pain or like a vegetable. He suffered enough when Mother died because no one would make any decisions. I want him to be sure to know that I died this way. Do you promise me?'

I agreed to do anything she asked, marvelling at how beautifully organized she was.

'Now you'll be able to start the book on Michael X,' she said. 'Take about a month to get over this and then start writing. But mind you don't dedicate the book to me - I don't want to be associated with that horrible man.'

I decided to tell her that I had dedicated *The Cricket Conspiracy* to her, which would be published shortly. The book was about the trial of Peter Hain, the anti-apartheid demonstrator who had been charged with conspiracy. Jean was fond of Peter and admired his tenacity.

'Tell me what you've said about me?'

Finding it too much of a strain to speak, I wrote on a piece of paper the inscription I intended: 'In Memory of Jean Humphry: Always a Campaigner.'

She read this and smiled at me in appreciation. 'That's very nice,' she said.

Jean had always stipulated that she wished to be cremated and have her ashes scattered in an unmarked spot. She made one additional request as she asked, 'I want you to plant a Peace Rose in the garden for me. Remember the big one we had in the front garden in London - it was the loveliest plant I ever had.'

Her state of mind and gracefulness helped me through that vivid morning although occasionally I could not help but break down and cry. She did not weep at all.

'You really must control yourself, darling,' she rebuked me. 'This is all for the best. We can't alter what's going to happen and I'm quite happy. Of course I don't want to leave you but I can't take any more of this cancer. I'd rather die today in peace of mind, and enjoying your presence and love in my own home than in

111

some grim hospital ward after being knocked senseless with drugs for a couple of weeks. This is the best way, believe me.'

I knew in my heart that she was right – that this way it was for the best, and the knowledge relieved some of my agony. In the circumstances, this was the most perfect end attainable to our marriage. Jean had stoically endured tremendous adversity with such dignity for the past two years that it was now her turn to take the initiative. However, something was bothering her when she asked, 'Aren't you breaking the law in helping me to take my own life? Won't you get into trouble? I couldn't bear that.'

I had anticipated this and assured her that I had thought it all out. 'I shall say nothing about it. At any rate, the doctors looking after you know that you are seriously ill. Dr Gornall thought you would be dead by last Christmas so how can they question your death now? Even if they suspect something unusual, which I doubt, I think they are too intelligent and sensitive to the situation to make needless trouble.'

She persisted with her questions. 'But it *is* against the law, isn't it?'

I told her that it was a breach of the law but that such offences were rarely prosecuted.* 'I can handle it,' I assured her. 'We must not worry on this score. I've been able to think this over since last August and there is not the slightest doubt in my mind that if this is the way you wish to die, then it is my duty to help you.'

She was comforted by this and we resumed talking about our pleasant memories. Jean reminisced about the opening of the shop, furnishing the farmhouse, and helping Edgar and Vivienne make a success of their marriage. 'Viv has promised me that she will look after you,' she said. 'And I've told them all that they must accept whoever you choose. I've told them that it doesn't matter how soon you're married after I'm dead – I don't care if it's a month! Promise me that you will marry again.'

Through an abundance of tears which I could not control, I managed to nod an assent which meant that I would keep the promise.

'Stop crying,' she admonished me. 'Look at the time.'

It was just ten minutes before one o'clock.

*See Appendix.

112

I dried my tears and went out of the room to get the brew of sleeping pills and pain-killers which I had decided could be best mixed in a cup of coffee. The youngsters were all slumped in chairs in the breakfast room and I suggested, as I passed them, that they prepare themselves, adding, 'I think she's close to death.' I made two mugs of strong coffee with milk and into one I poured the potion. Putting them on a tray, I went back into the sick-room and placed Jean's on the table beside her bed.

'Is that it?' she asked.

I did not need to reply at all. I took her in my arms and kissed her.

'Good-bye, my love.'

'Good-bye, darling.'

She lifted the mug and gulped the contents down swiftly, leaned back on her pillow and closed her eyes. Within seconds she appeared to fall asleep and soon her breathing was slow and heavy.

I did not go into the garden as Jean had asked because I had to be sure that she was going to die. The thought that she might regain consciousness if the drugs were not strong enough was unbearable. I knew that Jean would be distraught if she came round and found that, after so well prepared a death, it had been a fiasco. We both knew that the time had come for her to die, that the disease had gone too far, and that there was no longer anything doctors could do for her.

After fifteen minutes she vomited slightly and as I wiped her mouth the panic mounted in me as I thought that the pills were not going to work. Perhaps she had not kept down enough of the drug? On a chair beside the bed lay two pillows which had been used to prop her into a sitting position; I decided that with the first stirring of life I would smother her with them. It did not matter to me that I would be breaking the law: this was an act which two partners owed to each other, a private death pact. Anyhow, I did not intend that anyone should know.

Jean lay breathing heavily as I continued my desperate vigil. However, she did not need further help. At 1.50 P.M., 29 March 1975, as I sat watching, she died peacefully.

APPENDIX

The Criminal Law Revision Committee of Britain in its 'Working Paper on Offences Against the Person', published in August 1976, reports as follows:

Aiding and Abetting Suicide

Although suicide itself is no longer an offence, a person who aids, abets, counsels or procures the suicide of another is liable to a maximum penalty of fourteen years' imprisonment under Section Two of the Suicide Act, 1961. This offence was recommended by us in our Second Report (Command 1187). By our terms of reference we had to assume that it should continue to be an offence for a person to incite or assist another to kill himself. We felt it was open to us on the present offences against the person reference, however, to recommend, if we thought it right, that the offence under section two be abolished.

As in the case of manslaughter by reason of a suicide pact, prosecutions for offences under section two are rare. Two types of cases may be distinguished. The first class of case is where one person persuades another to commit suicide. The persuasion may be by a person who stands to gain financial advantage or other benefit from the other's death. Although suicide is no longer an offence, we think it is a serious matter if one person persuades another to take his own life. We are unanimous in agreeing that

115

it should continue to be an offence. The second class of case is where one person assists another to commit suicide, for example, by buying a quantity of aspirin for the other to take. We considered whether there was any distinction to be drawn between this type of case and the first class of case. It is arguable that it is less serious to help someone, who had decided to commit suicide, to do so than to persuade someone, who had not decided to do so, to take his own life. However, having regard to the present legal position in regard to euthanasia, the majority of us think that assisting a person to commit suicide should continue to be an offence. Any difference in the seriousness of these two types of case can be reflected in the sentence.

In our view (with a minority of members dissenting), the maximum sentence of fourteen years' imprisonment at present provided by section two of the Suicide Act 1961 should be retained in order to cover the most serious cases. We favour also the continuation of the necessity for the consent of the Director of Public Prosecution to the institution of proceedings for an offence under section two as provided by section two (four) of the 1961 Act.

WIDENER UNIVERSITY
WOLFGRAM
LIBRARY
CHESTER, PA.

116

Derek Humphry was born in Bath. He has been a journalist for over thirty years, starting as a messenger boy in Fleet Street. He now works for the *Sunday Times* and is the author of several books. Ann Wickett, an American who came to Britain in 1973 to read for a Ph.D. in English Literature, is his second wife.